MORE THAN JUST A BABY

A Guide to Altruistic Surrogacy
for Intended Parents and
Surrogates

Sarah Jefford

SURROGATE & LAWYER

First published 2020 by Indie Experts
PO Box 1638, Carindale
Queensland 4152 Australia
indieexperts.com.au

Published by Indie Experts Pty Ltd
www.indieexperts.com.au
QLD 4051, Australia

ISBN: 978-0-6489060-0-1 (pbk)
ISBN: 978-0-6489060-1-8 (ePub)
ISBN: 978-0-6489060-2-5 (mobi)

This book is dedicated to intended parents and surrogates who want to focus on the best interests of their children, and have a positive and amazing surrogacy experience.

CONTENTS

INTRODUCTION

My story

Many years ago, my husband and I decided to have children, and after several years of trying, we turned to IVF. We went through an IVF cycle and I produced 18 eggs. We created fifteen embryos and I underwent seven embryo transfers before falling pregnant with our first son, Archie, in 2009. Two years later we decided to try for another child, and while saving for another round of IVF, we fell pregnant naturally with our second son, Rafael, in 2012. We decided after his birth, that our family was complete.

While my partner and I felt that we were very much finished creating our own family, I had some sadness that I would never be pregnant or experience childbirth again. I donated eggs to several families and one of them went on to have a child with my help. Soon after donating my eggs, I explored the possibility of becoming a surrogate.

My husband and I talked about surrogacy extensively, before eventually meeting the couple who would become our intended parents in 2016. As a team we had counselling, underwent psychological assessments, obtained legal advice and had various blood tests and police checks before gaining approval for the arrangement. What had begun as a gestational surrogacy arrangement (where the surrogate carries a baby not related to her) later became a traditional surrogacy arrangement (where the baby is the genetic child of the surrogate). I conceived a baby and gave birth to their daughter in 2018.

Surrogacy has brought so much love and joy not just to the intended parents, but to me, my partner and our children, as our families are now forever intertwined and bonded.

Surrogacy has been one of the most amazing experiences of my life. I am so proud of what we have achieved as a team and the love we share with each other and the children in our families. But I have also seen surrogacy arrangements go sour, and often it is because the relationship between the intended parents and birth parents falls apart. Surrogacy is complex, and there are many opportunities for things to go wrong. As a lawyer and a surrogate, I have observed many surrogacy teams both flourish and struggle, and that has led me to write this book.

If we are to grow our families through surrogacy and donor conception, we need to make informed decisions that protect the interests of everyone involved, but most importantly are in the best interests of the children – those who are already here, and those who will be in the future.

I am a surrogacy lawyer and I assist surrogacy teams across Australia with their arrangements. I also blog about surrogacy and donor conception, and produce the *Australian Surrogacy Podcast*. I advocate for education and information about altruistic surrogacy in Australia, to empower intended parents, surrogates and their families and promote the best interests of children born through surrogacy.

About this book

This book is for anyone considering surrogacy, in Australia or overseas. It is for intended parents, surrogates and their partners, and donors. When I considered becoming a surrogate, I was dismayed by the lack of reliable information available and struck by how self-reliant intended parents and surrogates needed to be. I often wondered where the guide book was, to help us navigate the process and give language to our experiences. Surrogacy in Australia is not common, and finding accurate information and resources is important to ensure that we are not isolated and can access support from the community and professionals when we need it.

As with all good guides, this book should be read in conjunction with other resources, including those listed within the book. I would urge anyone interested in surrogacy to connect with other intended parents and surrogates. I am grateful for the community around me and recommend that you seek out other intended parents and surrogates for information and support. Research widely; surrogacy is a unique experience and no two surrogates or intended parents will have the same experience.

While every effort has been made to check the details of the information in this book, legislation is often reformed and updated. This book does not qualify as legal or medical advice; you should consult a lawyer and your own medical practitioner and clinic for specific advice that applies to you and your particular circumstances.

Surrogacy is a journey not a destination. You may enter the process with a range of expectations, fears, doubts, hopes and dreams. In the best case you will leave with an extended family and a wonderful experience to treasure for the rest of your life. And most importantly, my hope is that you also leave a legacy for the children born through surrogacy that is a story of love and long-lasting friendship.

CHAPTER 1

What is surrogacy?

A surrogacy arrangement is where a woman carries and births a child for another person or couple, who are the intended parents. After the birth, the baby is raised by the intended parents.

In Australia a surrogacy arrangement is altruistic, meaning it is unpaid and uncompensated. Commercial surrogacy is illegal across Australia; a surrogate must not be paid or receive a reward or fee for being a surrogate.

Do I qualify for surrogacy?

The intended parents must qualify for surrogacy. There must be a social or a medical need for surrogacy. This means that the intended parents must not be able to either conceive or carry a baby themselves, or to do so might be risky. A person who has a uterus must obtain approval to proceed with a surrogacy arrangement from their medical practitioner before proceeding to surrogacy. If you have a uterus and have suffered with infertility, surrogacy is one option, but it must be the last option. For many women and heterosexual couples, infertility can be treated in a number of ways, including different treatment protocols or with donor eggs or sperm. Infertility is really unfair, but having a surrogate carry a baby must be the last option after exhausting all other options available to you. If your doctor has not raised the option of surrogacy with you, then ask them if it is something that you should consider. A medical need for surrogacy might also include a psychological need.

There are no other legal requirements for qualifying for surrogacy – it is simply whether you have a social or a medical reason to not be able to conceive or carry the baby yourself.

If you are considering surrogacy, your first step is to talk to your treating medical practitioner and seek a referral to a fertility specialist to discuss your particular circumstances and whether your situation is considered appropriate for surrogacy.

Types of surrogacy

There are two different forms of surrogacy which are both legal in Australia: gestational and traditional.

Gestational surrogacy

Gestational surrogacy involves a surrogate becoming pregnant with an egg from an intended mother or donor, and sperm from an intended father or donor. The surrogate is not the genetic mother of the baby she is carrying. This is the most common form of surrogacy, both in Australia and overseas.

Gestational surrogacy is more common now due to the advances and availability of fertility treatments, which enables the intended parents to create embryos with eggs from the intended mother or an egg donor. Many surrogates are more comfortable with gestational surrogacy as they do not wish to have a genetic connection with the baby they are carrying.

Gestational surrogacy can be more expensive than traditional surrogacy, as it requires the use of IVF treatment. For intended mothers, it offers the opportunity to share genetics with the baby, and also allows for genetic testing of embryos which can increase the chances of conception.

Traditional surrogacy

Traditional surrogacy involves a surrogate using her own eggs to conceive, with sperm from an intended father or a donor. Traditional surrogacy is legal in most states.

Though it is worth contacting fertility clinics to enquire about traditional surrogacy, many will not facilitate such an arrangement. This leaves artificial insemination (done at home) as the remaining option. However, while the conception is arranged in private, the parties must still go through the process of counselling and obtaining legal advice before conception and completing the legal requirements after the birth.

While traditional surrogacy may not often involve an IVF clinic, it is not something to pursue simply to save on expenses. It can be easier to seek an egg donor than to pursue traditional surrogacy in Australia as fewer surrogates are prepared to carry their own genetic child.

Surrogacy laws and regulations

Surrogacy within Australia is regulated by various state legislation, and also by the Commonwealth *Family Law Act 1975*. There are no uniform laws, which means each surrogacy arrangement can be unique in the detail. There are restrictions on advertising for a surrogate or to be a surrogate in most states. Of particular importance is that no one should be advertising a willingness to enter into a commercial arrangement, as to do so is illegal.

The surrogacy laws that apply are those of the state where the intended parents live, regardless of where the surrogate lives.

It is legal in most states for intended parents to be single or a couple, married or de facto, regardless of sexual orientation or gender identity. There are some restrictions that, at the time of writing, are the subject of law reform.

In many cases, it is a requirement for the treatment and conception to occur in the state where the intended parents live. This means that the surrogate and her partner may need to travel to the intended parents' state for any treatment.

This book does not detail the surrogacy laws in each state because the laws and regulations are often changing. For up-to-date information about the laws that apply to you, visit www.sarahjefford.com.

Common criticisms of surrogacy

I believe that a woman has the right to full bodily autonomy. That includes reproductive autonomy: the right to determine if and when she has children, how many, and the right to make decisions about her fertility and reproduction.

I exercised my bodily autonomy when I had my own children, and later to assist people with the donation of my eggs and as a surrogate.

Bodily autonomy is a key tenet in altruistic surrogacy arrangements in Australia and is one very big reason why we do not have commercial surrogacy in this country. But critics of surrogacy are often against all types of surrogacy, including altruistic. Common criticisms of surrogacy can be summarised as follows.

That surrogacy is akin to child trafficking, or 'baby selling'.

This criticism might be levelled at commercial surrogacy, which involves fees and contracts and the end result is a baby being handed over. Arguably, the criticism can also be directed at altruistic surrogacy; the fact that no money changes hands does not alter the fact that a baby is being handed over. In Australia, however, the child's rights are paramount. If a surrogacy arrangement goes badly, it is not enforceable; the child's rights will be the primary consideration when determining who should be responsible for them and where they should live. It is not possible to have a contract on a child in Australia. And while not perfect, the counselling and legal processes surrounding altruistic surrogacy demand that the parties consider the rights and interests of any child born through the arrangement.

That surrogacy contracts are oppressive and deny a woman her right to bodily autonomy.

Some critics liken surrogacy to prostitution in that it involves the commodification of a surrogate's body for someone else's purposes. Again, some of this criticism might be levelled at commercial surrogacy and particularly in circumstances where surrogates live in poverty and are contracted as surrogates, precisely because of the financial gain they will make for themselves and their families. Some of the contracts in those arrangements are offensive. Control of the surrogate's body and autonomy includes clauses that restrict her movements and require her to adhere to strict living conditions. To be fair, those scenarios are less likely in developed countries such as the US and Canada.

In Australia, where there is no fee or payment in exchange for a baby, the surrogate maintains her bodily autonomy. I emphasise to clients entering into surrogacy arrangements in Australia that the surrogate can determine the care she receives during pregnancy, and she can consent or withhold consent to any treatment, including termination of the pregnancy.

As for the argument that surrogacy is like prostitution, I say that women have a right to determine what they do with their bodies, and this includes surrogacy and sex work. If we are really worried about the exploitation of women (as surrogates or sex workers) then we should be focused on regulating the industries and supporting all women to make informed and empowered choices for themselves. Stigmatising or criminalising surrogacy or sex work does not safeguard women's rights.

There is no right to a child; people who are unable to conceive or carry a child themselves must reconcile themselves to being child-free.

I agree with the critics in part on this issue. There is no right to a child. We are socialised from an early age to believe that when we grow up, we should find a partner, settle down and have children. Most people do not spend time considering this in depth, nor consider whether having children is something they really want. The nuclear family is considered the ultimate goal of anyone of child-bearing age.

While I do not believe anyone is *entitled* to a child, I still carried for a couple who wanted one. Because I maintain that I have the right to bodily autonomy and reproductive autonomy, and the rights of the child were maintained as paramount. The child I carried is loved and cherished by her parents and all her family.

Cancelling the critics

We may never be able to reconcile criticisms of surrogacy with the reasons why we do it. They may never convince me that all surrogacy is bad, and I will never convince them of how amazing it can be. My belief is that women should be empowered to make informed decisions, even if we do not agree with their choices.

Critics of surrogacy often rely on anecdotal evidence of a few women who had poor surrogacy experiences. It would be fantasy to assume that all surrogacy is good and all outcomes are positive. It is disappointing that a few stories should serve to promote the abolition of surrogacy altogether, or to bolster the opinions of those who claim we are all being exploited. I am not looking at surrogacy through rose-coloured glasses; I know that most surrogacy is imperfect, and that we can all do more to make it better. The rights of the child should be at the forefront of our minds, and surrogates must maintain bodily autonomy if we are to protect the integrity of altruistic arrangements. People should recognise that no one is entitled to a child, no matter the hardships they've confronted – it's not fair, but having a baby is not a right. And ultimately, it is the right of every woman to determine whether she carries a baby for someone else, and we should provide an appropriate framework to ensure her rights are protected. Abolishing surrogacy is not the answer; regulation is the key.

Critics of surrogacy argue that a child has a right to remain with its birth parents, and that a surrogacy breaks a primal bond between the birth mother and the baby, to both their detriment.

These same critics believe a woman should have the right to conceive a child that she intends to raise herself. The choice to grow your own family is not questioned. The problem, it seems, is the idea that a woman might want to conceive, carry and birth a child, but not raise them herself. So then, is the problem that pregnancy and birth are risky, or is the problem that the baby will not remain with the birth mother? Critics accept that we can have children if and when we choose, but only if we are determined to raise them ourselves. The conceiving and carrying is OK, but society expects women to raise the babies they birth and are critical when they choose not to.

The practice of surrogacy is quite old in some cultures, including the practice of *whāngai* in Māori culture, whereby a child is birthed by one woman and raised by others in the community as determined by what is best for the family and community as a whole.

The traditional version of family in our Western culture is that women must carry and birth children and then raise them with absolute devotion and tenderness. And yet, so many families do not fall into that stereotype and we know that families, women and mothers come in many different forms.

I am birth mother to the baby I conceived as a surrogate. I conceived and birthed her with the intention that she would be raised by her dads. My expression of bodily autonomy, of motherhood, is as her birth mother. I expressed my reproductive autonomy, of being able to conceive and carry her, and I expressed myself as a fertile woman, to be her birth mother. I never wanted to raise her. That is the version of motherhood I did not plan for. I never intended on mothering her. When critics of surrogacy claim that the rightful place for a child is with the birth mother, it is to deny that motherhood and mothering comes in many forms, and that the best place for a child is not necessarily with the person who birthed them or with those who they share a genetic connection with. A woman is capable of more than just motherhood in the traditional sense of birthing and raising children. When critics claim that all surrogacy is exploitative, what they are really saying is that there is only one, correct way to be a mother, and that is to keep the baby and raise it herself. I find that particularly reductive and patronising.

We know that genetics alone do not make a parent. I think about the sense of obligation and ownership that exists in many parent–child relationships, and how they are often not in a child's best interests. Being fertile and heterosexual are not qualifiers for being good parents, and we know that children raised in other families are healthy and well-adjusted regardless of their genetics and family creation. I am a birth mother, and by far the best thing I ever did, and did for her, was to hand her to her fathers so that they could be her parents. My act of selfless, unconditional mothering for her was not to raise her but to give her to her dads.

CHAPTER 2

Becoming a surrogate

Can I be a surrogate?

Many women who are thinking of becoming a surrogate may assume they will be eligible, often because they consider themselves fertile and have had smooth pregnancies and births of their own babies. It is worth exploring whether you are a good candidate for surrogacy, particularly before you offer to carry a baby for intended parents and get their hopes up.

Is there an age limit?

In most states, you need to be over 25 years old to be a surrogate. There are no legal restrictions on the upper age limit, but clinics often apply an upper age limit of 52 or 53, which is the average age of menopause. A post-menopausal woman can be a surrogate, so it is worth speaking to a medical practitioner about your situation if you are in your late forties or post-menopausal.

Do I need to already have a child?

In many states, you need to have had your own child before you can be a surrogate. This is not a legal requirement in New South Wales or Queensland at the time of writing. There is an argument that in order to provide informed consent to be a surrogate, you must have experienced pregnancy and childbirth already. If you have not had your own child previously, you might like to access counselling to talk through the possible impacts and consequences of pregnancy, birth and surrogacy.

Do I need to have completed my own family before becoming a surrogate?

Lots of people will declare that you must have *finished* your own family before becoming a surrogate. There are no legal requirements or restrictions on whether you must have finished your own family. Many surrogates continue to grow their own family after the surrogacy; no one can stop you from choosing to do that. You need to weigh-up the risks to yourself in any pregnancy, and whether you are willing to accept the risk that a surrogacy pregnancy may impact your ability to have more children. For example, if the surrogacy pregnancy results in complications that leave you infertile, will you be OK with not having more children? That is an individual decision for you and your partner; no one else can make that for you.

What if I'm single?

You do not need to be married or de facto yourself – there are many single women who are surrogates. Just like all surrogates, you should consider the support systems you have in place for yourself and your family before proceeding.

If you have been married and are now separated, you may need to consider finalising your divorce before entering into a surrogacy agreement. You need to seek legal advice about your particular circumstances, as each case is different. Being married at the time of entering into the arrangement should not impact on the treatment, but it can have implications for the parentage order (see chapter 14).

Do I have to live in the same state as my intended parents?

The surrogacy laws that apply will be those of the state where the intended parents live. You should get some advice about your circumstances before proceeding if you live in a different state to the intended parents.

Which type of surrogacy is right for me?

You can be a gestational surrogate, using an egg from the intended mother or a donor, or a traditional surrogate, using your own egg. There are different considerations and laws that apply to both, and you should get advice before proceeding with either option.

Does my physical health matter?

Many surrogates will feel that they are fit and healthy and able to carry a pregnancy, but you will need to speak to a doctor and obtain clearance before proceeding. In some states and clinics there are specific requirements and a doctor will need to approve you before you can become a surrogate. You can start the conversation with your treating doctor to see if there are any physical reasons why you should not carry.

There are no laws that say you can or cannot be a surrogate based on your physical health, but the doctor will consider your past pregnancy and birth history, your overall health, your age and your BMI. Some doctors may ask that you are under a certain BMI before trying to fall pregnant. Other health conditions might not disqualify you if the doctor is satisfied that you and the baby would not be at risk.

If you are considering becoming a surrogate and are wondering whether you would be approved, you should speak to your own GP first. The fertility specialist treating the intended parents may need to approve you as a surrogate before you can proceed. It is important to speak to your GP before offering to be a surrogate for someone, in case there is any medical reason why you would not be approved.

Could my mental health history stop me from becoming a surrogate?

Many surrogates worry that a previous history of mental ill-health will disqualify them from being a surrogate. A history of anxiety or depression will not disqualify someone, but it is an individual decision and one to be made with your support system and the surrogacy counsellor. A condition that is likely to be triggered by surrogacy, pregnancy or birth could be a reason for hesitation. The professionals involved will want to know that you have a good support system and access to mental health support during the process and beyond. Minimising your previous history or current mental health is not in your interests – much better to be open and upfront and prepare yourself for the times when you need support.

Like everything in surrogacy, it is important to do your research before jumping in.

What about the surrogate's partner?

There are a few heroes in the story of surrogacy – but none more unassuming than the surrogate's partner. The surrogate partners may not ask to go down this path, and the rewards for them are few and far between. But their support is crucial, and without it most surrogates would not be able to carry a baby for someone else. There is no 'i' in surrogacy – it's a team effort, and the surrogate's partner is as much part of the team as the surrogate herself.

So, what is required from partners to support the surrogacy arrangement? Well, firstly, they need to be engaged enough to make a decision as a couple on whether it is right for their family. Often, the surrogate raises the idea and reads and researches surrogacy and how it works. As the idea grows in her mind, she will want to discuss it with her partner to see what they think. Some partners may be against the idea entirely, while others might be open to the idea of it but need more information and time to think about it before committing. Partners should engage enough to find out information to understand why their partner wants to be a surrogate, and the basic legal and counselling requirements and processes. At this stage, they might also like to consider counselling with a surrogacy counsellor to discuss the big issues together and clarify what they want from the experience. Counselling can also assist them to determine if surrogacy is right for their family, and if so, how to find intended parents that are right for them.

I considered that, while egg donation was my decision and the impact on my husband was likely to be minimal, surrogacy needed both of us to be fully committed for it to go smoothly. My deal-breaker, which I kept in mind during the process and the pregnancy, was that my relationship with him had to remain intact beyond surrogacy. If he was unhappy, uncomfortable or unsupportive of anything, then we could not proceed until that issue was resolved. My relationship with him was more important, to us and our children, than the surrogacy itself.

From a legal standpoint, surrogate partners must be involved in the process because when the baby is born, the law presumes that the partner is also the legal parent. This includes being named on the original birth certificate. It means that the partner has to sign the surrogacy agreement. Post birth, they need to sign an affidavit supporting the parentage order. Their support cannot be blasé or token – it's all-in, or not at all.

In practical terms, the requirements of the surrogate's partner include the following:

- Attending counselling and undergoing a psychological assessment
- Obtaining legal advice and signing the surrogacy agreement
- Undergoing blood tests – this will depend on clinic policy, but it is often required that surrogate partners be tested for STIs prior to any embryo transfer.

The most important support that the surrogate's partner will provide is during pregnancy, birth and the fourth trimester. This includes practical support such as picking up the slack around the home and with the children during times the surrogate is tired, unwell or heavily pregnant, and when she is attending medical appointments. This can have an emotional and physical impact on the partner, and on the relationship between them and with the intended parents. If the partner is not fully supportive and involved in the surrogacy, the tough times during pregnancy can lead the partner to resent the surrogacy and the intended parents.

Partners often worry about the impact of surrogacy on their family and the surrogate. There are physical and emotional risks with any pregnancy, let alone doing it all for someone else. Partners understandably worry about how those risks impact on their family. It is important for the partners to access support themselves, and to talk about these fears during the surrogacy counselling. I'm a great advocate for counselling for everyone, simply as part of any wellness plan, and it can be crucial as part of a positive and smooth surrogacy journey.

The partners are also impacted by the surrogacy in other ways. They often receive similar questions to surrogates, which can be intrusive and even upsetting. Questions about how they feel about their partner carrying a baby for someone else, as well as all the usual curiosity about how a surrogate can possibly give away a baby. Partners are not immune to the effects of intrusive or curious questions, and it is important for the team to prepare themselves for how they might support each other and respond to people outside the team.

CHAPTER 3

Costs of surrogacy

One of the first questions from anyone pursuing surrogacy is how much it will cost. For altruistic surrogacy in Australia, there are so many variables depending on individual circumstances, so it can be hard to give an exact answer to that question.

Intended parents should expect to cover the expenses incurred by the surrogate and her partner in relation to the surrogacy arrangement, pregnancy and birth. You will need to get specific legal advice about what costs the intended parents must cover under the relevant state legislation, as it varies.

You might expect the surrogacy in Australia will cost anywhere from $15,000 to over $100,000. Most intended parents will spend somewhere in the middle of those figures. The major variable is the cost of fertility treatment, which will depend on what sort of treatment you require, and the success of any treatment and when the surrogate falls pregnant. Many intended parents will have already spent significant sums on fertility treatments before turning to surrogacy.

The costs you might expect

Fertility treatment
This will depend on how many cycles are required, whether donor eggs or sperm are required, and the success of the treatment. Read further to find out more about Medicare and rebates.

Legal advice
Lawyers' fees might be an hourly rate or a fixed fee. Lawyer fees vary considerably and depend on a number of factors, including whether you need a written agreement. You should compare quotes beforehand and seek out lawyers who specialise in surrogacy law. Some lawyers who do not practice in surrogacy law will charge for the time spent researching the law. Intended parents need to cover the cost of their own legal advice as well as that of their surrogate and her partner.

Counselling and psychological assessments
Some fertility clinics provide counselling as part of their service, while often it is conducted externally and incurs a separate cost.

Pregnancy and birth
Surrogates are eligible for Medicare and public healthcare, just as if they were having their own baby. Medical costs that are not covered by Medicare need to be covered by the intended parents. This includes private health insurance, private healthcare and hospital fees. It also includes medication and treatments that might be required during the pregnancy and birth and postnatal period.

Parentage order

After the baby is born, the intended parents need to apply to court for a parentage order to recognise them as the legal parents and to change the birth certificate. This can involve lawyers, and further counselling.

A breakdown of examples of expenses incurred for surrogacy

Pre-surrogacy expenses

- Counselling
- Legal advice
- Medical assessments, blood tests, screening of surrogate
- Police checks if required
- Psychological assessments
- Prenatal supplements
- Health, life and disability insurance for the surrogate.

Surrogate expenses

- Childcare for times when she attends appointments, or is unwell, or is recovering from birth
- A cleaner for times when she is unwell, or heavily pregnant, or sore. Some surrogates suffer with back and pelvic pain in early pregnancy, so do not assume that a cleaner is only needed in the last trimester or after birth
- Gardening or home maintenance
- Maternity clothing
- Medication, including prenatal supplements, pain

25

medication, medication for pregnancy symptoms such as heartburn and low iron

- Holistic therapies such as massage, naturopathy, acupuncture or chiropractor
- Travel and accommodation for surrogacy and pregnancy appointments
- Food and meal delivery, particularly if the intended parents are not local to the surrogate
- Lost income for during pregnancy and around the time of the birth. There are legal limitations on how much leave is covered, but if she has a medical certificate then the intended parents should cover her lost income.

Pregnancy expenses

- Private health insurance premiums
- Healthcare not covered by Medicare. Most surrogates will access public healthcare which is covered by Medicare. Any out-of-pocket expense must be covered by the intended parents
- Doula, birth support or private midwife expenses. This will vary according to each surrogate's preference
- Birth photographer – highly recommended but not compulsory. You can read more about birth photography in chapter 11
- Ultrasounds. Some pregnancies have one or two ultrasounds, while others have more depending on the care provider and the health of the pregnancy.

Post-birth expenses

- Pain medication
- Post-birth medical treatment for surrogate and baby
- Lost income of surrogate and partner
- Travel expenses for surrogate family – this may include taxi charges if she is unable to drive post-birth.

Medicare

As previously mentioned, surrogate pregnancies are treated the same by the health system as any other pregnancy. Surrogate pregnancy healthcare can be accessed under Medicare, and this includes public health and hospital care. Any out-of-pocket expenses after the Medicare rebate has been applied should be covered by the intended parents.

Medicare rebates are not available for surrogacy IVF treatment; however, this is applied differently depending on individual circumstances. If the intended parents are accessing IVF treatment prior to pursuing surrogacy, they may be able to access Medicare rebates.

Will the surrogate ask for money?

Surrogacy is altruistic in Australia. That means that payment of any type, or a reward or material benefit, is illegal. That includes cash payments as well as large gifts like a new car or paying for an overseas holiday.

I used to be offended by the question 'How much were you paid?' because I know that I didn't do it for money, and neither do the surrogates I've spent time with and advised over the years. Some intended parents worry that they should expect to pay their surrogate 'under the table'. I want to uphold the ethics of altruistic surrogacy and the suggestion that money must be changing hands is upsetting.

But then I think maybe we should talk about it more openly. And that talking about it might raise the standard that we expect of surrogacy in Australia. Because intended parents need to be reassured that there is no 'catch' and that they do not have to secretly pay their surrogate in order to pursue surrogacy in Australia.

Sometimes the question is because they themselves cannot imagine going through pregnancy and childbirth, giving away the baby, and not receiving some sort of payment. I used to think this was just cynicism. I do not think this means that the person is suggesting that being kind and selfless is something they cannot imagine. For many people, pregnancy and child-birth is hard. For many intended parents, pregnancy and birth has been traumatic and painful. They cannot imagine doing it for someone else without payment. As a friend once told me, 'You could not pay me $100k to carry a baby for someone else.' And when I consider her experience of pregnancy and birth, I understand.

For surrogates, pregnancy and childbirth are relatively easy and enjoyable, and they do not expect a negative experience in a surrogacy pregnancy. They like being pregnant, but probably feel that their family is complete and want to give the opportunity of parenthood to someone else.

If I was to give advice to any intended parents who are

worried that they may be asked for money or payment of any kind by a potential surrogate, then it would be to back away, fast. If she is asking for money or some sort of generous gift, she is not in it for the right reasons, and you will likely not have a positive journey. If you are OK with paying for surrogacy, then there are commercial surrogacy options overseas. Paying a so-called 'altruistic' surrogate undermines the standard we have established in Australia and dilutes the generosity of her actions. If you cannot trust her not to ask for money, then I would argue that you should not trust her to carry your baby.

On a positive note, have faith. While there may be a few instances where someone will expect or ask for payment, it is not the norm and the majority of women who are surrogates are not paid and do not expect payment. Trust that this is the case, and hold yourself to that standard. Do not expect other people to behave in an underhanded way, and maintain your own integrity throughout. Talk to other intended parents and surrogates about their experiences – the community will hold people accountable if we think anyone is motivated by money or seeking to avoid the legal framework.

CHAPTER 4

What to consider when seeking a surrogacy arrangement

Overseas surrogacy

When you are researching surrogacy options and agencies and joining the community, you may feel overwhelmed and unsure about the process. There are a few factors to keep in mind as you do your research and assess your options.

Be aware of people in the surrogacy industry and community who receive kickbacks for recommending services.

Intended parents may be forgiven for thinking that everyone they talk to about surrogacy has their best interests at heart. If someone seems kind, knowledgeable and generous, surely they only want to help you have a baby, right? But surrogacy is an industry like any other, and not everyone who seems helpful is looking out for your interests.

There are overseas surrogacy agencies who pay commissions to consultants and brokers who refer intended parents to them. Consultants come in many forms – they may also be intended parents, fertility specialists or lawyers. You should be wary of people preying on vulnerable intended parents, and particularly people not declaring that they are receiving commissions from the organisation they are referring prospective intended parents to. This is a conflict of interest, if they are making money for referring you to an agency and not telling you about it. You need to question whether their interests lie with you, or with the agency.

To help you make informed decisions when considering overseas donor and surrogacy arrangements, consider the following advice.

Cast the net wide

Research far and wide about all the surrogacy options. There are lots of agencies and clinics in various countries, and not all of them will be the right match for you. Surrogacy is a marathon, not a sprint, and you should commit several months to researching the options and gathering information to make a final decision. Best-practice arrangements involve known donors and a relationship with your surrogate. The agencies should be able to provide a detailed breakdown of their fees and expenses, and candidly answer your questions about surrogate recruitment and screening, fees, insurances, timelines, processes and contracts. If they avoid your questions, they may not be right for you. If their promises seem too good to be true, they probably are.

Ask the question

If you are meeting with someone to discuss donor and surrogacy options, be assertive and ask if they are receiving commissions, including co-marketing fees or benefits from any other organisation. If they say, 'You should try Agency ABC,' you should ask, 'What is your relationship with Agency ABC? Do you have a business relationship with them? Do you receive money for referring people to them?' Some consultants only work for one agency or clinic, and they will openly declare their interest. My rule of thumb is that if someone is upfront about their interest, then they are more likely to be honest with you. They should not be interested in your business 'at all costs' and should be happy enough to see you go elsewhere if they are not the right match for you.

Go direct to the source

One option is to avoid consultants and brokers altogether, and go direct to the source. Agencies and clinics will offer video conference consults direct with them, which means you know that no one is benefiting from your business but them. It is worth emailing them direct and asking to meet with them.

Watch out for the self-serving criticism of competitors

If someone is criticising agencies or clinics, consider whether they have a vested interest in you not choosing those agencies or clinics. Ask the question. Go to the source and ask them the question too. View criticism with a pinch of salt and use it to inform how you research that option further.

Speak to other intended parents – and ask the question

Other intended parents are an amazing source of information and have often done a tonne of research themselves. They can provide reassurance about the process and advice about the challenges and successes. But some intended parents may also receive commissions. If they are referring you to their agency or clinic, ask them if they are receiving a benefit for the referral. They should be declaring their interest to protect yours.

Domestic surrogacy

What to consider in seeking surrogacy team-mates

The relationship between the intended parents and surrogate is lifelong – it is worth taking the time to know each other and build the friendship. When we consider surrogacy from the perspective of the child born through the surrogacy arrangement and the children already here (the surrogate's children and the intended parents' children), we should be ready to commit to a lifelong relationship with each other. Before seeking intended parents or a surrogate, you should be clear about your expectations for the relationship and the sort of people you want to be friends with for the rest of your lives. A child born through surrogacy is best served knowing and having a positive relationship with their birth family and knowing that the adults involved made well-considered decisions with the expectation of being in each other's lives for the long-term.

This is, arguably, a higher bar than what we set for fertile couples who are intending to have children. But surrogacy is more complex and demanding than traditional family creation, as it involves more than just the two people who wish to be parents and their genetic offspring.

Here are some things that surrogates and intended parents should consider before they seek a surrogate arrangement.

- What are our expectations for a relationship with our surrogate/intended parents?
- Would we like to be local to each other, or is distance not a problem?
- For surrogates and their partners – do we have preferences for particular intended parents? A gay couple? A heterosexual couple? Singles? Cancer-survivor? A couple with a child looking to have another child, or a couple with no children?
- Would we prefer a family member or friend, or are we willing to meet new people and form a long-term relationship?
- What are our views on religion, and teaming up with people who might have a different faith to us?
- What are our values on termination of pregnancy, and teaming up with people who might have a different view to us?
- Are we financially secure enough to pursue surrogacy? For intended parents – do we have a plan for how to afford surrogacy?

- How do we communicate, with each other, and with other people in our lives? Could we improve the way we communicate?
- How will our family and friends react to surrogacy? Do we need to address any concerns or questions with particular people?
- Will our workplace/s be supportive?
- Should we access counselling before seeking a surrogate or intended parents to help us decide if surrogacy is right for us?
- Are both members of our couple committed to the process and relationship?
- Do we have a set timeframe or any deadlines?
- Have we thought about how we as individuals and as a team will respond to and manage disappointment, pregnancy loss or unsuccessful pregnancy attempts?
- Do we have other commitments that need priority or to be changed to accommodate surrogacy?
- Do we have any set ideas about medical treatment during pregnancy?
- Do we have hard and fast ideas about pregnancy and birth options and healthcare?
- What do we think about vaccination, and does it matter whether we share the same views as the other parties?
- Is there someone we can talk to about these issues – other intended parents, surrogates, counsellors, lawyers, donors
- Have we read widely and considered the possibilities and consequences before speaking to other potential team members?

Make contact with a surrogacy counsellor

An experienced surrogacy counsellor can help you prepare for the journey ahead, and can even help you decide if surrogacy is right for you. If you are the intended parents, you may have had a long and difficult journey to get to surrogacy. If you are a surrogate, you may be excited to get started. Regardless of which side you are coming from, you need to know whether you are ready for the journey ahead. A counsellor can help you to prepare and give you clarity about what to expect.

Creating embryos

While you are researching, talking to professionals and getting to know other people in the community, you should also consider what options are available to make embryos. If you need an egg donor, you might want to look for one before searching for a surrogate. Embryo creation takes time. Some clinics cannot make embryos before a surrogate is available, due to the state laws, so it is worth seeking advice about your specific circumstances to find out the best way forward. Many surrogates will ask whether you have created embryos and will be interested in how prepared you are to move forward in the process. (See chapter 9 for more on embryos and donors.)

CHAPTER 5

Finding each other: overseas

International surrogacy

While altruistic surrogacy in Australia is growing, it is not common. For many intended parents, international surrogacy will be an option they explore.

The laws

Commercial surrogacy is illegal across Australia. Most states, however, do not prohibit its residents from pursuing commercial surrogacy outside Australia. In Queensland, New South Wales and the ACT, it is a criminal offence for intended parents to enter a commercial surrogacy arrangement even overseas.

Exploring the options

If you are considering surrogacy overseas, there are many options and issues to think about. I recommend that you do your research, from various sources, and consider what is right for you and your family.

Nothing in this book should be taken as a recommendation or otherwise of any of the international surrogacy options. The more research you do, the better, for your interests and that of your future child.

When pursuing surrogacy overseas, you should think about your own values and ethics, and what the things are you will and will not compromise on. There are some crucial things to consider when engaging in international surrogacy.

Is the surrogate financially secure?

Surrogates should be not be primarily enticed by financial reward. Unfortunately, when there is little to no regulation, surrogates can be exploited by carrying a baby for intended parents they may never meet, for very little money. Surrogates are also the first to be punished when the laws change or authorities become involved.

If the surrogate is not financially secure, or if her primary motivation for being a surrogate is for financial reward, then consider whether you can be sure that she is not vulnerable to being exploited. Women in some overseas jurisdictions are recruited on the basis that they are desperate for money and therefore vulnerable to exploitation.

Does the surrogate speak English, and can she read, write and communicate effectively in English?

There are cases of surrogates signing surrogacy contracts despite having little to no literacy. One way to ensure that she understands what she is consenting to is to talk to her yourself – in English. Consider also how effectively you will be able to engage and communicate with her about all the intricacies of the process if she does not have proficiency in written or spoken English.

Will you be able to have a direct, open and engaged relationship with the surrogate?

Some surrogacy agencies overseas expect that the intended parents and surrogate will not have a relationship at all – but you should demand better, for yourself and your future baby. Unless you have direct contact with your surrogate, you cannot be certain of the information provided by the agency or clinic, and you cannot be certain that she is being looked after.

Does the surrogacy agreement provide for the surrogate to retain at least some bodily autonomy and to make decisions about her body?

Contracts that treat her like a commodity and completely remove any autonomy are exploitative and not in her interests nor those of any child born through the arrangement. Clauses such as that the surrogate will terminate a pregnancy upon request of the intended parents should be avoided. Many teams will reach agreements about pregnancy termination, but it should not be the sole decision of the intended parents. Likewise, clauses that restrict her eating and lifestyle habits may only serve to make her feel that the intended parents do not trust her, and this is not good for the relationship.

If you are pursuing surrogacy overseas, explore the options in countries that have well-trodden, well-regulated frameworks that protect the rights of the child and surrogate.

Read reviews from other intended parents, and do your research. Be aware of the track record of countries with bad reputations with surrogacy.

Some countries are better regulated than others. More regulation is preferable for protecting the best interests of the baby, the welfare of the surrogate, and the interests of the intended parents.

Cheaper is not better

A fast, cheap way to a baby is not likely to be an ethical, safe way to create a family. If you are focused on the cheapest way to make a baby, you are taking significant risks with your family. I understand – surrogacy is expensive. But if you are committed to maintaining an ethical approach and supporting the interests of the baby and the surrogate, then it is worth the investment of time and money to get it right.

Watch out for flashy sales pitches and offers that seem too good to be true.

It is really easy, and cheap, to create a website with fancy graphics that makes promises of a baby (or two). Do not rely on the agencies or clinics to tell you the hard truths – why would they, when it might mean you go elsewhere? Do your research. Ask other intended parents about their experiences. Ask if the people referring you are making money from the referral. Do not believe all the promises and glossy pictures.

International surrogacy options

When you are considering surrogacy overseas, you may become overwhelmed with the options and processes and getting to grips with the laws surrounding international surrogacy. I cannot recommend a particular option or country, but there are organisations around that can help, and representatives from agencies and clinics who will happily tell you about their services.

Before travelling overseas to pursue any options, you should get legal advice about your rights and responsibilities and the processes overseas and for returning to Australia with baby.

The United States of America has well-regulated and established surrogacy options in most states. Commercial surrogacy is legal across most of the US; this means that the surrogate is paid a fee on top of having her expenses covered. Getting into and out of the US is usually smooth for intended parents. There are many clinics and agencies willing to assist you to find a surrogate and a donor/s if you need.

Canada has an altruistic model of surrogacy, similar to Australia but is not as limited in options for finding a surrogate. Surrogates are not paid to carry a baby, but they are reimbursed for expenses.

There are agencies and clinics in Canada who can recruit surrogates and match them with intended parents. Intended parents travelling to Canada can expect a smooth journey in and out of the country.

Ukraine is another option for commercial surrogacy. Intended parents should be cautious not to accept at face-value any guarantees or options that seem too good to be true. Surrogates and intended parents are not encouraged to have an ongoing relationship, and there may be language barriers that you need to overcome. Recent media suggests that surrogates and children may be exploited. Intended parents travelling to Ukraine can expect to be there five to 12 weeks post-birth while they wait for travel documents.

Other options

I have many clients asking about other options like Kenya, Greece, Georgia, Mexico and Colombia. I cannot say anything definitive about any of those options but advise you to exercise caution and careful consideration of obstacles and concerns.

Make sure you are operating within strong legal frameworks.

Many countries have little or no regulation or laws about surrogacy. This means that agencies can say 'it is not illegal here' – but that doesn't make it a good option. Good, robust legal frameworks supporting surrogacy are what you should be seeking. A lack of surrogacy laws means you take significant risks when you rely on it not being illegal.

Ongoing availability, knowledge and contact with the birth mother are important

Will your baby be able to contact their birth mother and have a complete knowledge of their own identity? How will the circumstances of their conception and birth potentially affect your child as they grow older and want to know about how they came into the world? Make sure the arrangement you adopt has transparency and encourages ongoing contact.

Safe and easy travel is crucial

You need to satisfy yourself that you can travel in and out of the country and leave with your baby in good time. I've heard many stories of intended parents being stuck in their destination country for weeks and months, unable to leave because they cannot obtain papers to travel to Australia with their baby. This is rarely the fault of the Australian authorities. If you are seeking to save money by going to an unregulated country, you may find that you spend more money trying to return home and having to support yourself and your baby while trying to leave.

Online resources for international surrogacy

You can join Facebook groups dedicated to Australians travelling overseas for surrogacy. You should find other intended parents who are at different stages of the journey to seek their support and share information. Groups are available for most current international surrogacy options.

CHAPTER 6

Finding each other: Australia

Domestic surrogacy

The quest to find a surrogate or intended parents can feel daunting and may seem impossible. Many intended parents have traversed this road before you and will have experienced the same feelings.

If you have been advised to pursue surrogacy to grow your family, you can start searching for a surrogate. Intended parents outnumber women who are willing to carry a baby for someone else.

Surrogacy in Australia is a bit like dating. And just like dating, it takes time and commitment for it to work. Most people would not consider marrying after the first date; consider the relationship with your surrogate as a similar long-term commitment. The parties need to be friends and have built sufficient trust for it to be a positive journey. Surrogacy is not just about making a baby – it is about growing families and friendships. Altruistic surrogates are not paid to carry a baby; their reward is entirely in the giving and the ongoing relationships they have with the family they've helped create.

Finding a surrogate in Australia is challenging and it takes time. There are lots of learnings, growth and value in the journey.

There are surrogates that have preferences for carrying for a gay couple, or a woman who has survived cancer, or someone with no children. Likewise, some surrogates are keen to support a single intended parent. The difficulty in Australia is not the preference; it is the lack of women willing to be surrogates. Half of Australian surrogates are known to the intended parents already – family or friends. The other half met their intended parents through social media and forums. Being single is not a barrier of itself to finding a surrogate.

Tips for finding a surrogate in Australia

Share your story

Share your story with family and friends and someone may come forward.

This might seem like a strange way to find a surrogate, but it can work. Many surrogacy arrangements in Australia are through existing relationships – that is, through friends and family members. Surrogates will often have considered being a surrogate for friends or family but not known if anyone needed one. Many intended parents will share their story in an email or social-media post to their loved ones and offer to talk to anyone who wants more information.

You may think that there is no one in your friendship circle or amongst your family members who could, or would, carry a baby for you. It is still important to share your story with your loved ones so that they have the opportunity to support you. Many people still believe that surrogacy is not legal in Australia, so by sharing your story you are helping to destigmatise surrogacy and donor conception, which is important for other intended parents, surrogates and particularly for children born through these arrangements.

While you might think that no one close to you will offer to carry for you, you will never know unless you are willing to talk about it. By sharing your story, you may also be starting many more conversations. I know of surrogacy arrangements that have started from conversations at the hairdressers, in the workplace, between neighbours and at school pick-up. If you are anxious about what to say, perhaps write a draft or think of the main messages you want to convey, and have someone proof-read it. Some ideas for what you can write in your post or message include:

- An update on your family and relationship, and what has been happening in your life that has led you to want to grow your family.
- That you need some help to grow your family, and the reasons why, if appropriate.
- Why growing your family is so important to you.
- That you have been reading and researching options for surrogacy (and egg donation, if necessary).
- Some information about surrogacy in Australia – that it is legal and altruistic – and where they can read more about it.

- Your reasons for telling your story and what you hope to achieve.
- An invitation for people to ask questions and continue the conversation.
- A statement of thanks for their support.
- You might like to include photos of yourself in the post or email.

There are several state laws prohibiting advertising for a surrogate. Be careful that your story is just that – that you want to have a child and your reasons why you need someone else to carry for you. Be careful not to say anything that might look like an advertisement. Some states allow for advertising, and you can refer to www.sarahjefford.com for more information.

Join an online surrogacy community

There are Facebook groups and forums you can join to meet other intended parents and surrogates. Below are a few you should try.

The Australian Surrogacy Community on Facebook is a social group of intended parents and surrogates from around Australia. It is well moderated and the community is supportive and generous with information. There are also regular catchups in many states which are organised through this group. I met my intended parents through this group, as lots of teams do.

Egg Donation Australia is another Facebook group and membership includes altruistic egg donors and egg recipients around Australia.

The *Australian Surrogacy Podcast* shares stories from

surrogates and intended parents who have been where you are and have generously shared their experiences so that others can benefit.

Connecting with a surrogate

It is all very well for me to give you advice about finding a surrogate, when really the challenge is *connecting* with a surrogate to the point where you can agree to enter into a surrogacy arrangement. Intended parents outnumber surrogates in Australia and so, even if you are a member of the right Facebook groups and forums, it can still seem impossible to find a surrogate you like and trust enough to start your journey with them.

I know that putting yourself out there as an intended parent, on social media, is scary and daunting. You are sharing the most vulnerable and intimate details of your life with virtual strangers. You need to see any potential relationship with a surrogate as authentic and reciprocal. Aim to connect with a woman and her family on many levels, not just about whether she will carry your baby.

Surrogacy is a journey, not a destination. Expect it to take a long time. Many surrogacy journeys take two or more years from meeting each other to having a baby. If your timeline is much less than that, you may need to consider other options outside Australia. You must invest in relationships if you expect altruistic surrogacy to work, and that takes time.

My advice when looking to connect with a surrogate is to be your authentic self. Surrogates want to know you and your story.

It can be exciting to embark on the road trip to a baby. Everyone gets a bit of 'baby lust' and can lose sight of the bigger picture. You might feel really ready to have a baby and know that you and your partner have thought this through and are committed to each other and to parenthood. But would you make a baby with someone you have just met, or only known for a few months? That seems like a big leap – and a bit risky. Take your time, do your research and find the right people to build a life-long friendship with.

Surrogates talk to each other and may compare notes – they will know if an intended parent has sent an unsolicited message to another surrogate. Surrogacy relationships are like dating – and like dating, you need to be active, engaged, curious and courageous. You also need to be respectful, friendly, supportive and authentic. If you moved to a new town and wanted to make new friends, how would you go about it? Would you knock on strangers' doors and demand a friendship? Or would you hang out in places and at events where like-minded people hang out, and start conversations?

Within the Facebook groups, questions are often asked – how do we start chatting with a surrogate? How do we know which surrogates are available and willing to get to know us? Intended parents should be careful about sending a message to a surrogate without their permission. For surrogates to see and notice you, intended parents need to post and comment on other threads – be active and engaged. But surrogates also want to get to know you, beyond surrogacy. They want to know your story, how you came to be a couple, why you're pursuing surrogacy, what you do for a living, what you are passionate about.

That means being in it for the long haul. One post introducing yourself is unlikely to be noticed. But posts and comments that are curious and supportive are likely to be noticed. You need to put something into the surrogacy community if you want to take something from it.

Do not underestimate the power of a positive review. Many surrogates will seek counsel from their fellow surrogates, to see what they think of certain intended parents, or to enquire as to who the intended parents are in their local area. I met my intended parents after following the recommendations of another surrogate, because there was nothing so reassuring as the positive review of someone who had already spent time with them and could vouch for them. Make friends with community members – surrogates and intended parents – with the aim of having friends along for the ride, with an added bonus that those friendships may lead to a woman offering to be your surrogate.

My advice for finding and connecting with a surrogate includes:

- Be active and engaged on the forums, share your story and be supportive, kind and helpful within the community.
- Be authentic. You do not want to find a surrogate at the cost of your values or because you have presented yourself in a certain way that you cannot sustain. You want to connect with a surrogate that you can have a

lifelong friendship with, not just a woman who has a working uterus.

- Build your community. The surrogacy community is strong and supportive of those who contribute and participate. If you want to connect with a surrogate within the community, you need to contribute what you hope to get out of it.
- Make friends with people in the community. Do not make friends with the sole hope that they might carry your baby; make friends with lots of people in the community because those friends may help you find a surrogate, and because they'll be your cheer squad along the way. Follow the rules. Do not send unsolicited messages to surrogates. Do not jump on a new surrogate when she introduces herself. She will see right through it – and so will everyone else.
- There are local catchups in each state – picnics, brunches, dinners and coffee-catchups. These are all about community-building, but they're also really great for finding that cheer squad I mentioned, learning from others and finding support. You should seek out and attend the local catchup groups in your state.

CHAPTER 7

The process

The surrogacy process

1 **QUALIFY FOR SURROGACY**
The intended parents need to meet the criteria for surrogacy in their state.

2 **MEDICAL ASSESSMENT**
The surrogate attends a medical assessment by an obstetrician.

3 **COUNSELLING**
All parties involved have counselling about the surrogacy arrangement.

4 **LEGAL ADVICE**
The intended parents and the surrogate and partner obtain legal advice from two different lawyers.

5 **PSYCHOLOGICAL ASSESSMENT**
Some clinics and states require the parties to be psychologically assessed.

6 **APPROVAL**
The surrogacy arrangement is approved by the clinic or external committee before any embryo transfer can occur.

The surrogacy process in Australia is similar in all states, and applies to all arrangements regardless of how the parties know each other or their relationship with each other.

These steps are followed for surrogacy arrangements facilitated by a clinic. For traditional surrogacy arrangements not utilising a clinic, parties need to obtain counselling and legal advice prior to conception.

Counselling process

Counselling is a crucial part of any surrogacy journey, and not just because it is required by law. Counselling provides an opportunity for team members to work through issues together and separately, maintain their mental health and support the team as individuals and as a group. If you are focused on building and maintaining a long-term relationship with each other, for your own sake as well as that of any children involved, counselling should be a priority for everyone.

There are legislative requirements for what the counselling sessions need to cover. Your counsellor should be registered with the Australia and New Zealand Infertility Counsellors Association (ANZICA) and experienced with surrogacy and donor conception. There are ANZICA Surrogacy Guidelines, which you can access online, that provide guidelines for counsellors to ensure they cover the important issues for each surrogacy team.

The guidelines were drafted with four key principles in mind, based on the Surrogacy Matters Parliamentary Inquiry 2016.

1. The best interests of the child
2. The surrogate's ability to make free and informed decisions
3. Ensuring the surrogate is free from exploitation, and
4. Legal clarity about the resulting parent–child relationships.

Once the team is approved for their surrogacy arrangement, counselling takes on a more supportive role for the pregnancy attempts, pregnancy and birth. My advice is that there is no such thing as too much counselling, and every team member should access support for their journey and mental wellbeing. Surrogates should have access to regular counselling and intended parents should ensure that they allow for counselling as an ongoing expense.

Many states require the parties to undergo post-birth counselling and relinquishment counselling. These are procedural requirements for the parentage order. However, post-birth counselling is crucial for the team and individuals to be able to debrief the birth, and support them through the fourth trimester (the three months after pregnancy) and beyond.

Legal advice

The parties to a surrogacy arrangement, whether it is traditional or gestational surrogacy, must obtain independent legal advice. This means that the intended parents have one lawyer, and the surrogate and her partner have a separate lawyer. The parties often require a written agreement, which can be drafted between yourselves or by one of the lawyers.

You can read more about the legal process and implications of entering into a surrogacy agreement in the next chapter.

Other requirements

In addition to counselling and legal advice, some clinics and states will require other checks and balances before entering the arrangement. These can include psychological assessments, police and child welfare checks, blood tests and STI checks.

The Patient Review Panel in Victoria and the Reproductive Technology Council in Western Australia have their own processes for approving surrogacy arrangements that are separate to the IVF clinics. You should refer to their websites and get advice about how those processes impact on your circumstances.

Things to consider when starting the process beyond the formal requirements

While the law, regulators and clinic operators may have a formal process for surrogacy, there are other components to consider as you begin and progress through the process.

Building the relationship

Altruistic surrogacy is all about the relationship. Whereas commercial surrogacy might be considered transactional and involves the payment of a fee, altruistic surrogacy is relational. I mean no disrespect to commercial surrogacy relationships, but the dynamic is fundamentally different. Surrogates are not paid, but they rely on the relationship with the intended parents. The reward and the fulfillment of surrogacy is seeing the intended parents meet their baby and become parents, and having an ongoing relationship with them.

Surrogacy relationships really are like no other relationship. A woman is carrying a baby with the intention of another person or couple raising the child. The intimacy is similar to that of pair-bonded couples. We are conceiving a child with people we are not in a pair-bonded relationship with. We are crossing invisible lines of intimacy and trust, normally reserved for pair-bonded couples. Surrogacy relationships are some of the most complex relationships we might experience as human beings.

Surrogacy involves a redefining of friendship and family. Expectations that we might have of our friends or family members are completely different to expectations in surrogacy relationships. Surrogacy counsellor Katrina Hale says that intended parents may worry that the surrogate might not hand over the baby, and the surrogate may fear that the intended parents will use and abandon her. These fears can manifest in a relationship push-pull situation.

What are some of the things we can do to build the relationship and prepare ourselves for the journey ahead?

Build a relationship outside of surrogacy
Spend time together getting to know each other, without talking about surrogacy. Spend time with each other's families and friends. Invite the other parties to social gatherings with your

other friends. Try not to separate surrogacy from the rest of your life. Surrogacy will, at some point and over a long time, feel all-consuming. There is no way to sustain it as an element separate from the rest of your life.

Spend family time together

Too often, surrogacy relationships are based on getting together for surrogacy appointments. Family time together – cooking together and for each other, visits to the playground, watching a movie, walking the dog, even holidaying together – can build the relationship.

Setting expectations

To prepare for the surrogacy journey, teams should commit some time to discussing expectations, prior to speaking to a lawyer or counsellor. This should lead on from building the relationship and help you prepare for the challenges ahead.

When travelling down the surrogacy path, the most important part is the relationship between the surrogate (and her partner, if she has one) and the intended parents. And rather than just hoping that everyone is on the same page, it is much better to commit some time and energy to setting expectations and building the relationship and trust between you. The list of issues that you need to discuss is endless – but can arguably be divided into five main categories.

On the following page is a detailed breakdown of topics for discussion. These lists were developed with the other surrogates during the Surrogacy Sisterhood Retreat. While these lists are not exhaustive, they might assist in developing your own list and start conversations in your own team.

Before conception
Communication – frequency, methods
Timeframes
Legal advice – which lawyers and when
Counselling – clinic or private and when
Childcare arrangements for surrogacy appointments
Meeting up and spending time together
When to tell others of the plans
Social media sharing and tagging
Number of pregnancy attempts
Managing disappointments and hurdles
Embryo creation and quality
Geographical logistics
Political views
Taking time out from surrogacy
Mental health support

During pregnancy
Communication
Vaccination (of surrogate and intended parents)
Termination of pregnancy
Coping with pregnancy loss
Birth and parenting classes
Genetic and diagnostic testing
Hospital and healthcare provider choice
Health and fitness

Help at home for surrogate family
Childcare
Spending time together
Social media sharing and tagging
Announcing pregnancy to others
Counselling and mental health support
Attending appointments
Scans
Asking for help

Labour and birth

Birth plans – hospital, home
Type of birth, pain relief
Support persons, doula/private midwife
C-section arrangements – who will be in theatre
When will the surrogate tell the intended parents she is in labour
Childcare arrangements
Travel to hospital
Birth photographer
Who 'catches' the baby
Skin-to-skin
Cord clamping
Colostrum, milk and feeding
Rooms and arrangements at hospital
Leaving hospital
Surrogate's family to visit
Placenta
Announcing the birth to others
Social media sharing and tagging

Sarah Jefford

Fourth trimester and beyond
Vaccinations
Medical treatment
Cuddle time with surrogate
Contact arrangements – visits, frequency, logistics
Photographs
Social media sharing and tagging
Timeframe for intended parents to return home (if not local)
Milk and feeding
Paperwork for birth registration and parentage order
Counselling and mental health support
Ongoing future contact
Language and roles – Aunty, Birth Mother, Tummy Mummy
Asking for help

Financial arrangements
Intended parents' capacity to fund the surrogacy
List of expected expenses
Surrogate and partner's time off for appointments
Payment arrangements – reimbursement, EFT, bank card access for surrogate
Communication – appointing 'spokespersons' for each couple

You may access a free template, Setting Expectations, via my website (see Additional resources on page 166), that you can use as a team to write your own.

Money talks, but what if we do not like talking about money

It is a fact universally known that altruistic surrogates do not like to talk about money. Surrogates do not like asking for money, and they would rather spend their own money than burden the intended parents. Surrogates may feel that any talk about money can undermine the altruism of the gift that they are giving. And let's be honest, no one really likes talking about money. But in surrogacy arrangements you have to grin and bear it, because you have to talk about money at some stage.

The number-one rule of altruistic surrogacy is this: the surrogate should never be out-of-pocket. Altruistic surrogacy does not mean free. Surrogates are already putting themselves and their family's wellbeing at risk by carrying a baby for someone else – they shouldn't be financially worse off for doing it. While there are legal frameworks for what expenses should be covered, the rule of thumb should be that if it is surrogacy, pregnancy or birth related, the intended parents should be covering it. If it's an expense that the surrogate would not have incurred if she were not pregnant with someone else's baby, then the intended parents should be covering it.

So how do you have the conversation if she will not talk about it? Well, in some ways you need to take it out of her hands. Make it as easy as possible for her, and make sure she is never out-of-pocket. The easiest and least stressful option to ensure your surrogate is not out-of-pocket is to provide her with access to funds ahead of time. Many teams find the easiest way to manage expenses is to provide the surrogate with a bank card with access to dedicated funds for surrogacy expenses. This way the surrogate can use the card for expenses, there is no need for reimbursing after she has spent her own money, and there is a record in the intended parents' bank account of any expenses she has incurred.

As for the tough conversations about what everyone agrees is to be covered and how much, these are best had as a team, and both in and out of counselling. Do not rely on the counselling to cover it all – utilise the counselling as a starting place for ongoing conversations. Recognise that it is awkward. And in particular, recognise that the surrogate is likely to minimise her needs and will likely say 'it's fine' and 'do not worry about it'. The intended parents need to be proactive about money – do not wait for the surrogate to ask for money or request a certain expense. The chances are, if she wants a new maternity bra, she will spend her own money to buy it. The intended parents need to be assertive enough to insist that she spend their money on those expenses, and not take no for an answer.

Surrogate partners can also play a role in the money conversation. They are one step removed from the pregnancy and might find it easier to have hard conversations with the intended parents about expenses. The surrogate does not want her altruism undermined by money conversations, while her partner can make sure there is money secured for a cleaner, for example, and that her request for maternity clothing is met. She can then feel comfort knowing that the conversations are being had, but that she can focus on herself and the baby.

Here are my five tips to ensure money does not kill the relationship:

1. Have pre-conception agreements about how money stuff should be dealt with.
2. Have a linked card for the surrogate to utilise to pay bills etc. so she doesn't have to ask for money or reimbursement.
3. Nominate a communication avenue to discuss money. Have it in writing, email or text, to avoid confusion.
4. Nominate a spokesperson from each team to discuss money.
5. Keep it unemotional and business-like.

Social media and sharing

You may be surprised (or not) to discover that something as simple as social media can cause a rift in surrogacy teams, particularly if the expectations and rules are not established early on. Many intended parents want to keep their journey relatively private. They may have had a journey of infertility that makes them vulnerable and need to keep updates about growing their family to a small circle of intimate friends and family. When we share stories of infertility or grief, inevitably someone has words of advice that may be unhelpful and unwelcome. People can make rude comments and ask intrusive questions, without real-ising the impact or the hurt the person hearing those comments is feeling.

Surrogates, on the other hand, may be excited to share the story, because being a surrogate can feel isolating. Sharing on social media can widen their network of support to include other surrogates.

When it comes to sharing our stories on blogs, social media, or in the wider media, it is important that the team has open discussions about expectations and agreements beforehand. If one party is more open to sharing the surrogacy journey than others, then compromises can be reached about what information is shared and when.

To help you determine what is right for your team, you might like to discuss the following:

1. What information and updates are we all comfortable sharing on social-media platforms?
2. What are our privacy settings? Are our updates for close family and friends, or for everyone in the world?
3. Are we tagging each other or naming each other in our updates?
4. Are we happy for other members to share more of our story on their own social media, even if we are not sharing?
5. Are we sharing photos of each other and our children?
6. What photos and details are we sharing of the birth and about the baby, and when?
7. When are we announcing the pregnancy and birth?
8. What other things are we sharing about the surrogacy? Can we share photos and stories in the future, or is there a time limit?

Engaging with the media

If you are approached or are approaching other media outlets, be careful that the entire team is happy with the angle and the form the story will take. Headlines that read 'Womb of Doom' and 'I Had a Baby With My Brother' are not meant to garner the support of readers; they are meant to shock readers into finding out more. Beware that once the article is online, it can have a life of its own and you cannot control the comments once it is shared a thousand times around the world. If the team is engaging with media outlets, make sure you agree on which photos are included and what information is shared. Understand that some people sharing and commenting will disagree with surrogacy for various reasons, and that the story itself could start conversations that do not have a positive angle.

Be prepared that there will likely be negative and ignorant comments on social media if your story is shared publicly. This can be hurtful, and even traumatic, at a time in your lives when you may feel fragile. Prioritise your wellbeing and safety, and switch off from social media if you need to. Trolls are not interested in changing their minds, but they will enjoy engaging with you to get a reaction. The majority of comments will likely be positive and curious, so consider engaging with them only. These stories can serve an educational purpose for the community, which can be a good thing if done well. Think about the messages you want to convey and stick with them.

If you are engaging with people on social media about surrogacy, perhaps stick with the following messages:

- Altruistic surrogacy is legal across Australia
- We all had counselling and legal advice before entering the arrangement
- We intend having an ongoing relationship with each other
- The surrogate is happy and recovering well from the birth
- Thank people for their kind comments.

Navigating challenges

Every surrogacy team will hit hurdles and face challenges during their journey. This can include unsuccessful pregnancy attempts, pregnancy loss, miscommunication and misunderstandings, disappointments and mismatched expectations. Setting expectations early in the relationship can avoid some of the challenges, as can accessing counselling at regular times during the journey. Surrogacy relationships are some of the most complex, intimate and extraordinary relationships we will ever enter, and it is no surprise that they can also be the most challenging. Expect it to be hard sometimes. As a surrogacy lawyer, there is only so much I can do to help teams through the challenging times. By far the better option is to involve a surrogacy counsellor, for individual and team support, both as a treatment and an antidote for the challenges.

CHAPTER 8

Lawyers and legal advice

Why do we need lawyers?

Many people are confused and sceptical when they discover that they need to engage two lawyers for the surrogacy arrangement: one for the intended parents and one for the surrogate and her partner. You may feel like you know enough about the surrogacy process and laws and that you do not need a lawyer. So, what is the good of a lawyer, and why do you need one for a surrogacy arrangement?

Firstly, engaging two lawyers for an Australian surrogacy arrangement is a requirement for a parentage order in all states. You cannot enter into a surrogacy arrangement unless the intended parents and the surrogate and their partner have obtained independent legal advice. 'Independent' means a lawyer that has only advised the intended parents or the surrogate, not both. The intended parents must have a lawyer, and the surrogate and their partner must have their own lawyer. The intended parents pay for both lawyers. However, paying the bill does not mean the lawyer is answerable to the intended parents, who are not their clients.

Lawyers should consider and analyse agreements and arrangements from all angles and explore issues that you may not have considered. This is particularly true of an experienced surrogacy lawyer who has worked with teams through both positive and challenging journeys. It is a lawyer's job to reality-check your expectations and understanding of the consequences of entering into a surrogacy arrangement. Lawyers also have to certify that they believe that you have understood the advice they have given.

Written surrogacy agreements

Surrogacy arrangements are written into formal agreements between the surrogate and her partner, and the intended parents. The primary function of the written agreement is to provide evidence of the parties' intentions to enter a surrogacy arrangement, which is required as part of the application for the parentage order.

Most states require surrogacy arrangements to have a written agreement.

A written agreement is not enforceable, other than where a surrogate might need to claim costs and reimbursement for expenses incurred during the surrogacy.

A written agreement can help ensure everyone is on the same page and there are less likely to be conflicts or misunderstandings.

Written agreements should cover the requirements of a

surrogacy arrangement, such as counselling and legal advice. They can also cover agreements about other matters, such as:

- Pregnancy and birth care options
- What costs the intended parents have committed to cover
- How the intended parents will reimburse their surrogate for costs
- How the intended parents will support their surrogate and her family in times of need
- How the parties will communicate with each other
- How the parties might resolve issues and conflict as it arises.

Why surrogacy agreements are not like contracts

The elements of a basic contract include (1) an offer, (2) acceptance, (3) consideration (usually money) and (4) an intention to create a legal relationship. For example, you offer to buy a car for $10,000. The owner of the car accepts your offer; you provide $10,000 as payment (consideration), in return for the car. Both you and the owner of the car enter into a legal relationship to exchange money for the car.

In altruistic surrogacy arrangements, the surrogate and her partner offer to carry a baby for another person or couple and the intended parents accept. But there is no real consideration. The intended parents might get a baby, and the surrogate can expect to have her expenses covered. All going well, the surrogate is rewarded for her good deed with lots of love and fuzzy feelings. And while the parties might intend to enter a legal relationship, surrogacy agreements in Australia are not enforceable, other than to ensure the surrogate's expenses are covered.

So if an altruistic surrogacy agreement is not like a contract, why would you write it as if it were a contract? In most states, a written agreement is required as evidence of the arrangement and is a prerequisite for a parentage order. There are no prescriptive lists for what should be in a surrogacy agreement, which means you can include things that are important to you and leave out things that you do not want.

A good surrogacy agreement should be written in good faith to a trusting relationship between the parties. The surrogacy agreement is a piece of evidence of what the parties' intentions and obligations are as intended parents, surrogates or surrogate partners. The signed agreement is used as evidence for the clinic before doing an embryo transfer, and later for the court when making the parentage order. It is not binding, other than as it outlines the surrogate's expenses and the intended parents' obligation to cover them.

Lawyers should be a positive influence on the process – helping you understand the consequences of entering into the arrangement, and your rights and responsibilities. The relationships, however, will outlast any legal process. My advice is to focus on the relationship and building trust, and the counselling, to ensure you have a positive experience. Because at the end of the day, it will not matter what is written in an agreement; it is the relationships that are important.

I am always disappointed to hear that people have not had a positive experience with the legal agreement or the legal advice they have received, or feel that their lawyer over-serviced them and charged them a fortune beyond what is expected for a surrogacy arrangement. Often it is because there are aspects of the surrogacy agreement that seem to pit the parties against each other. Clauses that restrict, limit or prohibit the surrogate from behaving in a certain way, do nothing for the trust between the parties. It can be really damaging to their trust. Surrogates are doing an amazing, generous thing to carry a baby for someone else. If the agreement dictates how she must behave or provides her with a list of prohibited behaviours, her first reaction may be to think the intended parents do not trust her. And if they do not trust her to do the right thing by their baby, then perhaps they should not trust her to carry their baby at all.

Why are surrogacy agreements not enforceable?

The answer is both simple and complex and comes back to two primary concepts.

Firstly, the rights and best interests of the child are paramount. You might be thinking, *but surely the child's interests are best served if they are living with the intended parents?* Well, that might be the case, but it might not. And actually, it is a lot more complex than just a matter of handing a baby over to the people who are their intended or genetic parents.

If we make a surrogacy agreement enforceable, that makes it more like a contract than an agreement. If you make a surrogacy agreement enforceable, you elevate the interests of the intended parents above the rights and best interests of the child. A woman engaged as a surrogate in an enforceable contract will be forced to hand over a baby, not because it is in the child's best interests, but because she will face consequences for breaching the contract if she does not. And while it might be in the child's best interests to be raised by the intended parents, that is not a decision that should be determined by enforcing a contract against the surrogate.

The other reason why surrogacy agreements are not enforceable is that a surrogate retains her bodily autonomy throughout treatment, pregnancy and birth. 'Enforceable contract' and 'bodily autonomy' are mutually exclusive. A surrogacy agreement cannot be enforceable and still uphold the surrogate's right to bodily autonomy. She cannot, for example, be forced to undergo certain treatments, or a pregnancy termination, or to continue a pregnancy against her will. If you make surrogacy agreements enforceable, you are limiting a woman's bodily autonomy.

What happens if the surrogate keeps the baby or the intended parents will not take it?

If surrogacy agreements are not enforceable, the question remains: what happens if the surrogate decides not to relinquish the child? Or if the intended parents decide not to take the child?

The fact that a surrogacy agreement is not enforceable does not mean that a surrogate can simply change her mind and keep the baby. Nothing, when it comes to children and their care, is that simple. The Family Court has jurisdiction to determine what is in a child's best interests. If a surrogacy agreement goes awry, the parties can issue court proceedings and ask the court to determine what is in the child's best interests.

Evidence of a surrogacy agreement between the parties is important for the court to consider, but of itself it does not sway a court to make an order for the child to be handed over to the intended parents. The court is more interested in the particular circumstances of the case, including all the parties involved, and determining what is in the best interests of the particular child in the case in front of them. What this means is that no two cases are identical, and a finding in one case does not necessarily influence a judge to make the same decision in a similar case.

What we know is that a child has the right to know and be cared for by both its parents. Who is a parent is a matter of debate, particularly in a surrogacy arrangement. A child has a right to an identity, and that includes knowledge of and access to information about their genetic and birth heritage. DNA does not make a parent, but it is an important part of a child's identity. The court is also interested in the capacity of the parties involved to provide a caring, safe and positive environment for a child to be raised in.

In Australia, there have been very few cases of surrogacy arrangements going so badly that the courts needed to determine where the child lived and who raised them. As mentioned above, if it were to happen that the surrogate chose not to relinquish the child, the court would make an assessment on all the facts and circumstances to determine what is in the child's best interests.

If, on the other hand, the intended parents could not, or chose not to take the child after the birth, the surrogate and her partner would need to make a decision about the care of the child. Most surrogacy agreements will include the names of people that the intended parents have nominated to take the child if they were to pass away. The intended parents should update their wills to nominate guardians to care for their minor children in the case of their deaths. The surrogate and her partner might also raise the child themselves, or hand over the child to family members of the intended parents to raise. The surrogate and her partner could proceed through an adoption arrangement. No matter the outcome, there would be some legal process and recognition of the arrangements for the child's future care.

If the intended parents separate before or after the birth, they can and should continue with the parentage order process and make arrangements between themselves for the ongoing care and parenting of the child. Separation is not a reason for the surrogacy arrangement to fall apart. The parties are expected to proceed with the arrangement, regardless of their relationship status.

If the surrogate and her partner separate at any time, both will be expected to continue with the parentage order process, including providing their consent to the parentage order being made.

If one of the intended parents dies before the birth, the surviving parent can still take the baby and apply for a parentage order.

Surrogates will be anxious to know that the intended parents have made arrangements for the child's care in case of their deaths. Surrogates and their partners are not usually prepared for an additional child in their family. While the surrogate and her partner will have considered and appreciated the risks of entering into a surrogacy arrangement, the intended parents should ensure they have discussed the arrangements were they not able to take the child after the birth.

What happens if you proceed with surrogacy without going through the legal process?

The surrogacy laws and other laws surrounding children, adoption and parentage is complex. There are several laws that cover children, and the Commonwealth *Family Law Act* dedicates almost 200 pages to clauses addressing children's issues. There are also many cases that give us some insight into how the courts view issues of parentage and surrogacy, and what is to be considered when deciding what is in a child's best interests.

People often ask why they need to involve lawyers in their surrogacy arrangement. It's a good question, given that surrogacy agreements, even if they are in writing, are not enforceable. While making a baby is an emotional, human, and sometimes medical process, surrogacy is much more complex and involves a legal process. Transferring parentage from birth parents to intended parents is not a simple matter of a private agreement. In cases where the parties decide to make a baby and hand it over to other people to raise, there is a risk that it can be seen as an informal adoption (at best) and as human trafficking (at worst).

Sometimes, a woman will offer to be a surrogate for people she met online, and to do it cheap and easy without involving lawyers. The question must be asked: what is her motivation for avoiding the counselling and the legal process? If she is looking for 'cheap' or 'easy', her motivations may not be genuine, and intended parents take significant risks in proceeding with the arrangement. I would discourage anyone from pursuing an arrangement that is off-grid, without involving lawyers and counsellors. You must understand the risks, and consider the story you will tell your future child about their conception. If there are red flags flying, it is best to back away.

For gestational surrogacy, an IVF clinic will not proceed with the arrangement unless you have provided them with evidence that you have received legal advice and counselling.

So, what are the consequences of not following the process of a legal surrogacy arrangement? I've had a few cases which did not tick the boxes, and there are a number of consequences you should be aware of.

The intended parents will not be able to apply for a Parentage Order, transferring parentage from the birth parents to themselves. This means that the legal parents of the child will always be the birth parents.

The birth certificate cannot be changed. The birth mother will remain on the child's birth certificate. Only a Parentage Order can provide for the change of birth certificate. Unless the criteria of a surrogacy arrangement are met, the birth certificate cannot be changed.

Not having a birth certificate that lists the intended parents and child can lead to problems with Centrelink, Medicare, overseas travel, passports and enrolling the child in childcare and school. The intended parents may need to rely on the birth parents to sign any documents they need to exercise parental responsibility for the child. There are also risks that the legal parents – those named on the birth certificate – will be liable for child-support payments.

While the intention of the parties might have been to save money on lawyers (and counsellors), the end result will likely be more expense on lawyers and legal processes. If the intended parents wish, or are forced to apply for orders for parental responsibility (which is sometimes referred to as 'custody'), then the legal process to obtain such an order would likely be much more expensive than if the parties had done the surrogacy legal process before conception. The timeframe for obtaining parenting orders (as opposed to parentage orders, which are relatively easy) can be many months and several court hearings.

There is a risk the authorities may become involved and scrutinise why a child is being raised away from their birth family. Child protection authorities must ensure that children are safe and protected – if it comes to their attention that the birth parents are leaving their child with another family, it can look like abandonment or neglect, and worthy of investigation. Unless there is a surrogacy arrangement in place, the child protection authorities have the power to be involved in the family.

The courts can take a very dim view of an arrangement that involves parties giving a child to others without involving a formal legal process. A surrogacy arrangement is dealt with in the state courts, and as long as the parties have satisfied the criteria for a parentage order, it will be made and the birth certificate changed. The court hearing (where there is one) is ceremonial and celebratory, and the judge commends the parties on their love and commitment to the child. Where an arrangement has not followed the proper processes, the Family Court may become involved and it does not view those arrangements in the same light. Questions will be asked about whether the arrangement is in the child's best interests. The arrangement will be scrutinised not as an arrangement of love between the parties but, as one judge said in a case I was involved in, 'the commodification of women and children'. Questions may be asked whether there was an exchange of money between the parties.

You might be thinking that engaging in an informal surrogacy arrangement, avoiding lawyers and counsellors, is an easier option. After all, you all trust each other, right? But the laws are not there to make life difficult for you. They are primarily there to protect the rights of children, to ensure that women are not exploited, and to protect all the parties involved. And while there might be a lot of love and trust between the parties (or maybe it is just a woman on the internet promising you the world), the courts are full of people who once had loving and trusting relationships, arguing over what is in their child's best interests.

My advice is that getting sound legal advice about your arrangement – surrogacy, adoption, co-parenting or donor arrangement – is worth the investment. Family law is still evolving, and each situation calls for a unique approach. Investing in the right advice – before conception – is worth it at least to know that your future child will thank you for not cutting corners.

Gift giving

Commercial surrogacy is illegal, so it is important that a surrogacy arrangement be altruistic and that no commercial gain, reward or inducement is involved. But what does this mean if the intended parents want to show their surrogate their love and appreciation? What sort of gifts might be appropriate, and what might be considered a reward or inducement?

The laws can be interpreted very broadly, such that even the gift of a massage voucher or a bunch of flowers *could* be seen as a material benefit or reward for the surrogate. How then do intended parents look after their surrogate, support her through any treatment and pregnancy, and show their appreciation without crossing over into illegal territory?

The laws are designed to prevent commercial arrangements, involving women who are motivated to be surrogates for the promise of payment. The law is not designed to punish people who accept gifts of love, friendship, appreciation and support.

A good rule of thumb is to act as you would if you were giving a gift to a friend. Gifts that are not cash, such as massage vouchers, flowers, ready-cooked meals, movie tickets and dinner vouchers are unlikely to be considered by any reasonable person as an inducement or reward for surrogacy. And surrogates are unlikely to be motivated to go through the challenges of pregnancy simply for the promise of a free movie ticket or a massage.

Cash deposits into a surrogate's bank account are a bit trickier. It is expected and acceptable for the surrogate to be reimbursed for her lost of wages due to the surrogacy treatment, pregnancy or birth and postnatal period. Loss of wages might be paid into the surrogate's bank account in periodic or lump-sum payments. If this applies to your arrangement, you should ensure that the amounts deposited correspond to evidence of the lost earnings, such as payslips or a record of reduced work hours. Keeping accurate records of expenses and payments is important, in case you need to provide evidence that the arrangement was altruistic and not commercial.

For other reimbursements, such as the cost of prenatal supplements, or travel costs, consider direct payments to the clinic, or giving your surrogate a linked debit card that she can use to purchase pregnancy-related items. (See chapter 7 for suggestions on financial arrangements.)

Intended parents worry that if they give any gifts to their surrogate it could compromise the surrogacy arrangement and that the court could refuse to make the parentage order. The laws provide that the courts can refuse to make a parentage order if the arrangement looks to be a commercial transaction. And surrogates can be prosecuted if they have broken the law and received payment for being a surrogate.

If in doubt, you should contact your lawyer. My advice is to be kind, exercise common sense, and remember, if it looks like a commercial arrangement, it probably is. If it looks like a gift of love and friendship, it probably is.

CHAPTER 9

Conception

A right to know

Years ago, it was not uncommon practice for infertile couples to go to an IVF clinic and conceive a child with the assistance of an anonymous sperm donor. The clinic staff would tell the parents not to tell anyone – the child, or their friends and family – that they had the help of a sperm donor. Often, the parents were not given any information about the donor, and in many instances the records were not kept, or were destroyed.

Many decades later, we now know better and, hopefully, we do better. We know that at the core of any discussion about donor conception should be the interests of the donor-conceived person. While in the past we may have prioritised the privacy of the donor and the parents, we now know that that the donor-conceived person's interests are equally or more important. They have the right to access information about their donor and other donor-conceived siblings, including medical information. We also know that it is in their interests

81

to know from an early age that they are donor-conceived and to have the opportunity to meet and know their donor and donor-conceived siblings.

What we also know is that if a donor-conceived person is not told of their donor heritage, they will likely find out by accident or hearing it from people other than their parents. Over a third of donor-conceived people surveyed in Victoria found out they were donor-conceived via consumer-DNA websites such as ancestry.com

Unfortunately, there are places in the world where anonymous donors are not only available but still the norm. When children born through these arrangements grow up and want information about their donor or other donor-conceived half-siblings, they may hit dead ends or rely on DNA testing. Donor-conceived people are telling us now that this impacts on their emotional wellbeing and sense of identity. Many donor-conceived people report the distress they feel when they discover they have over 100 donor-conceived half siblings across the world.

Being told from a young age about their donor heritage and having access to information is important for a donor-conceived person's identity and sense of self. Keeping donor conception a secret can be harmful and is not in the best interests of a donor-conceived person.

How can we get donor conception right?

Use a known donor or an Australian clinic-recruited donor whose information is available to the donor-conceived person.

Utilise a donor who has adhered to family limits. Family limits are regulated in each state of Australia, and vary between five and ten families. Unfortunately, many donors from outside

Australia have often donated many times resulting in 100 or more donor-conceived offspring.

If you are seeking a donor overseas, insist on options involving a known donor. A 'known' donor does not have to be someone close to you but can be someone who is willing to be known to you and to the donor-conceived person and be available for contact in the future. Donors should consent to donor-linking in the future.

Avoid donor programs that involve strictly anonymous donors and poor regulation. Some programs insist, or are bound by the country's laws, to only facilitate strictly anonymous or no-contact donation.

Research donor conception, listen to the *Australian Surrogacy Podcast* interviews with people involved in the donor community, and read more about donor conception before making a decision.

Tell your child of their donor conception from a young age. VARTA (www.varta.org.au) provides resources and advice to donors and recipients about sharing the information with children. Celebrate the story and help your child celebrate their donor heritage. If it is shared with love and openness, it will be a positive experience for the child and will not be a source of shame.

Finally, remember that the interests of children are always paramount. It can be hard to focus on a child's interests when they do not yet exist, and when we are feeling baby lust. But, as one donor-conceived person advised, 'Celebrate the connections; do not fear them or create shame. These people are pivotal to who we are.' Celebrate your donor and their part in helping you grow your family.

Egg donation

Egg donation is one of those topics of interest in the media occasionally, and warrants a warm, fuzzy headline now and again, but good-quality information and resources are lacking. There are restrictions on advertising for an egg donor, and whether you are a donor or a recipient, finding the right information can be a matter of tenacity.

Egg donation in Australia is altruistic. Egg donors, like surrogates, cannot be paid for providing their eggs, but they must have their medical and out-of-pocket expenses covered.

How do egg donors and recipients meet?

In the case of egg donation, some clinics have access to an egg bank, but many do not. There are fewer egg donors than there are recipients in Australia. Egg donation, unlike clinic-recruited sperm donation, often involves recipients and donors meeting and getting to know each other before the donation occurs.

Are there criteria for donating eggs?

There are no laws determining the age or requirements for donors. Many clinics will have age limits and may also stipulate that the donor must have had their own child. However, many women are still donating in their late thirties, and many donors have never had their own child. An older donor is less likely to produce high numbers of eggs than a younger donor. You can expect that most might be reluctant to cycle with a donor in her forties.

are currently no government-run egg donor recruit-
ons. Most people find each other on forums, such as

Egg Donation Australia. There is also a Facebook group which you can join.

You might consider sharing your story with friends and family. Many recipients like the idea of a genetic link between themselves and their donor, so asking sisters and cousins is a good option. However, donation is not for everyone, and many women cannot fathom sharing their genetics beyond making a child with their partner.

What is involved in being an egg donor?

Egg donation involves counselling for the donor, her partner, and the recipients. The counselling should cover everyone's motivations and expectations for the donor-arrangement, including expectations for future relationships and for the child's relationship with the donor and their family.

The donor, their partner and the recipients will complete consent forms which includes details of how consent can be withdrawn. Donors and recipients should discuss their expectations for future use of the embryos, including in the case where the donor has died.

Once the counselling is completed, the donor can commence an IVF cycle, with the intention that the eggs collected will be fertilised with sperm from the recipient (or a sperm donor) and used by the recipients to achieve a pregnancy, either themselves or through a surrogacy arrangement.

Is a donor a parent?

This is a complex legal issue, but generally speaking, a donor is not a parent. At birth, the presumption is that the birth mother is the legal parent, and if she has a partner, they are also the legal parent. While the donor is genetically linked to the baby, genetics alone do not make a parent. The donor will have no parental rights or responsibilities, and while their information is recorded on the birth record, there is no parenting status that comes with that.

If you are considering a donor arrangement with a sperm donor and not involving surrogacy, you should get legal advice before going any further.

If you are an egg donor or recipient of donor eggs, there is no harm in obtaining legal advice about your rights and responsibilities. The clinic process and counselling should address the consequences and legal aspects of donation. Some teams like having a written memorandum or agreement that outlines their expectations for the future relationship, such as the amount of time the donor will spend with any children that result from the donation. An agreement might be useful to make sure everyone is on the same page.

Importing and exporting embryos

If you are considering surrogacy options in Australia and overseas, you need to consider where the embryo creation will take place and whether that will have an impact on your journey. There are restrictions on importing and exporting gametes (the male or female reproductive cell being either eggs or sperm) and embryos, both in Australia and in other countries, and you need to find out what those laws are before proceeding.

There are particular restrictions on importing and exporting donor gametes and embryos created with donor gametes.

It is generally easier to transport gametes and embryos created with gametes from the intended parents. There are also restrictions on transporting embryos if the donor was paid rather than altruistic, such as may be the case if you sourced a donor from overseas. Donors must also consent to having their information recorded, so that any child born from their donation can access that information when they are older.

If you are pursuing surrogacy overseas, you should consider whether it is better, easier or cheaper to create embryos in your destination country or within Australia. If you are creating embryos in your destination country, you should consider whether you may wish to bring the unused embryos to Australia and whether that will be feasible.

Factors to consider when creating embryos that you may seek to transport later include the following.

Whether you are creating embryos with the help of a donor and what restrictions apply in your state and the destination country for transporting donor gametes.

Whether the treatment you are seeking must occur within your home state. For example, some states require that the embryo transfer must occur within that state in order to qualify for a parentage order when the baby is born.

Whether you are eligible for the Medicare rebate if you create embryos in Australia and whether that makes it more affordable than creating them in your destination country.

Conception via traditional surrogacy

The complexities of genetics

Traditional surrogacy, where a surrogate becomes pregnant with her own egg and sperm from an intended father or a donor, is less common than gestational surrogacy in Australia. This can mostly be accounted for due to the availability of IVF, which allows intended parents to create embryos with their own gametes or with a donor.

Traditional surrogacy often involves home inseminations as the means for conception. Some clinics will facilitate traditional surrogacy, but unfortunately many are reluctant to be involved. Many IVF clinics have a policy that they will only assist with gestational surrogacy. Some clinicians believe that traditional surrogacy is risky because the surrogate will not hand over the baby – this is not based on evidence.

Intended parents may be interested in pursuing traditional surrogacy as it seems cheaper than gestational surrogacy – and for obvious reasons, if there is no IVF clinic involved. However, most surrogates are comfortable being gestational surrogates but are not comfortable with using their own eggs for the surrogacy arrangement. While the costs might be reduced due to the absence of IVF, cost should not be a primary motivator to pursue a traditional surrogacy arrangement.

Traditional surrogacy can seem simpler because you are combining the role of surrogate and egg donor. It can be more complex than gestational surrogacy because the birth mother is also the genetic mother of the child. This means that relationships extend well beyond the surrogacy itself, and the child will have a different relationship with the surrogate and her children because they also share genetics. Traditional surrogates, including myself, have found the experience enriching and rewarding, but also complex and challenging. There are very few traditional surrogates in Australia, and thus very little information or resources available.

If you are considering traditional surrogacy, either as a surrogate or intended parent, you might like to seek counselling, together and separately, to talk through the arrangement and the possible consequences.

CHAPTER 10

Pregnancy

Healthcare

Most surrogates have given birth to their own children and will have their own ideas and expectations about the sort of pregnancy healthcare they want for a surrogacy pregnancy. You should discuss these ideas and expectations as a team, and establish whether there are any inconsistencies or deal-breakers between you. Intended parents should undertake to do their own research and learning about pregnancy and birth.

While the surrogate can provide some information and insights into her experience, the intended parents should not rely on or expect her to educate them entirely. There are lots of resources available about pregnancy and birth, including books, YouTube videos and social media accounts dedicated to the subject.

From a legal and healthcare perspective, surrogacy pregnancies are no different to other pregnancies. The surrogate will be able to access public or private healthcare just as if she were pregnant with her own child. The decision whether to opt for public or private healthcare is entirely up to the team. Many hospitals will have their own policies about birth and post-birth care of a surrogacy arrangement. Metropolitan public hospitals may be under increased pressure due to volume and therefore less able to accommodate the team's requests and needs. On the other hand, private hospitals may be less inclined to support the needs of a surrogacy arrangement without charging for extra rooms after the birth.

Most hospitals will only manage a few surrogacy pregnancies in a decade. The chances of your hospital and your healthcare provider having supported a surrogacy pregnancy or birth in the last two years will be low. You will need to educate the healthcare provider and hospital, and advocate for the needs of your team.

If you are local to each other, intended parents should expect to attend most, if not all, maternity appointments with the surrogate. Many pregnancy appointments are boring and tedious. The team should discuss expectations about who attends appointments and how things are managed when it comes to making decisions during pregnancy. While the surrogate maintains her bodily autonomy throughout the pregnancy and birth, she will be keen to involve the intended parents in any decision-making that affects the baby. It is important for the intended parents to be involved in appointments, have access to the treating medical practitioners, ask questions and access information so they can make informed decisions with the surrogate.

Surrogate bodily autonomy

The two main facets of altruistic surrogacy in Australia are that the surrogacy agreement is not enforceable, and the surrogate maintains her bodily autonomy.

What does bodily autonomy mean?

A surrogate is just like any other person and can make decisions about her body just as any other person can. This is the case even when she is pregnant, and even when the baby is not intended to be raised by her and does not share her genetics. A pregnant person can determine what happens to their body, whether they receive a particular treatment or what food they eat. There are few limitations on a person's bodily autonomy, even if they choose to abuse their body with drugs or alcohol. In most states, a pregnant person can determine whether or not to continue the pregnancy, and how they are cared for in pregnancy and birth.

A surrogate does not lose her autonomy despite being pregnant with a baby intended for someone else to raise, or with their gametes. The team needs to discuss their expectations about what treatments she will have, and how she will manage the pregnancy. Will she drink alcohol, eat soft cheese, or go skydiving while pregnant? (See chapter 7 for a full list of expectations to discuss with the team.) There are no rules, but surrogates will generally treat the pregnancy and the baby much the same as if she were pregnant with her own child. Surrogates want the very best for the baby and will usually follow the recommendations of their treating medical practitioner. But if there are differences amongst the team about how the surrogate will manage the pregnancy, it is best to work through those issues prior to conception. Ultimately, the surrogate can make the final decision about anything that affects her body.

If you are an intended parent and you find it difficult to relinquish control to your surrogate, that is understandable. The person who is carrying your baby can make the final decision about whether she drinks, smokes or eats terrible food. You need to work through your anxieties about this prior to entering into the arrangement, and preferably with the support of a surrogacy counsellor. If you cannot relinquish control and trust your surrogate to take good care of your baby, then you should not proceed with the arrangement. It is important that your surrogate does not carry the burden of your anxiety during the pregnancy.

Termination of pregnancy

Where the surrogate's bodily autonomy can have the most impact is the issue of pregnancy termination. The team should talk about their views on termination prior to entering into the arrangement and discuss the circumstances where they may consider a termination. The team needs to understand each other's views and ensure they have discussed what may happen if they disagree. Ultimately, no one can force a surrogate to terminate a pregnancy, and neither can they force her to continue a pregnancy against her will.

While the surrogate's bodily autonomy is a legal matter, it is not a good idea to rely on lawyers to resolve any disputes between the parties. If the team is in disagreement about the surrogate's conduct during pregnancy, the primary concern should be about supporting the relationship between the parties and seeking counselling for support. Calling lawyers to resolve any disputes is unlikely to lead to a better outcome for the relationship.

Privacy and information-sharing during pregnancy

A surrogacy arrangement necessarily involves people sharing experiences with each other that would otherwise be reserved for the most intimate of relationships. Besides discussion about your views on pregnancy termination and whether the surrogate will drink alcohol during pregnancy, there are also discussions about the intimate details of the surrogate's menstrual cycle and the health of her uterus.

As we talked about in the previous section, a surrogate retains her bodily autonomy even when she is pregnant with a baby for someone else. She does not waive all her rights to autonomy, or privacy, simply by offering to be a surrogate. Most surrogates will be happy to share and discuss openly with her intended parents any information about the pregnancy and baby. But even when she provides her consent to sharing some information, it should never be taken as a sweeping consent to sharing all information.

As with every major issue in surrogacy, the team should discuss the topic of information-sharing and reach agreements about what information might be shared, how it is to be shared, and whether any team member wishes for some information to remain private.

Staff at IVF clinics might be challenged by the issue of privacy and information-sharing in surrogacy teams. The staff are used to sharing information about menstrual cycles, treatment and pregnancy with the woman they are treating. In surrogacy arrangements, the patients are also the intended parents, and the staff may be uncertain about what information about the surrogate's menstrual cycles, treatment and pregnancy can and should be shared with the intended parents. They may get it wrong – calling the intended parents with the results of tests done on the surrogate, and not asking the surrogate for permission to do so.

It is important to reach agreements about what is shared and how. To get it right, you might like to consider the following as a guide.

The surrogate maintains a right to privacy, and all information about her body, treatment she is receiving, her medical history and test results are her private information.

The surrogate should be provided with access to all information about anything to do with her body, health, treatment and results.

If there is information of interest to the intended parents, the surrogate must provide her specific consent to that information being conveyed to the intended parents or convey that information herself.

Unless the surrogate has provided specific consent to information being shared, then it remains her private information and should not be shared.

When providing consent to sharing information about the surrogate's body, health, treatment and test results with the intended parents, consideration should be given to whether the information is about the embryo, foetus or pregnancy, whether it is necessary or helpful for the intended parents to know, and whether they are able to understand the information.

Intended parents are not medical professionals and are not bound by professional or ethical standards of confidentiality. It is not appropriate that a surrogate's full medical history or records be provided to the intended parents simply because she is carrying their baby. She does not waive her rights to privacy, dignity and respect.

There should be no blanket consent on a surrogate's private information being provided to the intended parents in any circumstances.

Where information is being shared that is hard to understand or causes confusion or difficulties for and between the parties, counselling should be sought from an independent counsellor.

The surrogate can expect that some information be provided to the intended parents. For example, information about the embryo, and her readiness for embryo transfer. Later, that information might include details of the baby's growth and development and the surrogate's overall health. All that information should be considered in context of her privacy. Some ways to provide that information to the intended parents include:

- Inviting the intended parents and surrogate to attend appointments together
- Giving the information to the surrogate and allowing her to share that information with the intended parents

- Asking the surrogate if it is okay to tell the intended parents certain things about her health and the pregnancy and treatment
- Remembering that she is the patient and she has not signed over her rights to privacy and autonomy when she offered to carry a baby for the intended parents
- Seeking the surrogate's consent to speak directly to the intended parents.

Practical support for the surrogate family during pregnancy

Intended parents carry the pressure of wanting to be appreciative, supportive and caring for their surrogate and her family, and not wanting to be intrusive or overbearing. With that in mind, there are a few things that intended parents can do to support their surrogate and her family throughout the process. The ideas below are collated with the help of other surrogates and intended parents, but are just that – ideas. You and your team should sit down and consider the best way that the intended parents can support and be there for their surrogate (and that may be different if you are family, friends, local or interstate), and the surrogate family's particular needs.

First of all, the entire team might benefit from taking *The Five Love Languages* (www.5lovelanguages.com) test to determine what your love language is. The 5 Love Languages were developed by Dr Gary Chapman, who found that different people expressed their love in different ways. These are *words of affirmation, acts of service, receiving gifts, quality time* and *physical touch.*

The love languages are a great tool for understanding how each of member of a couple, or surrogacy team, gives, receives and communicates love. For me, for example, I think acts of service (doing things for me) and spending quality time with me are the best ways of letting me know that you care. Knowing each other's love languages can help the team determine the best way for the surrogate to be supported in the way she needs it. A surrogate who values acts of service may be more appreciative of homecooked meals delivered to her door than of a gift-wrapped box of chocolates.

You might also find that setting expectations (see chapter 7) for each stage of the surrogacy process helps in communicating expectations so that everyone's needs are met and there is less risk of conflict or misunderstanding.

So, with all that in mind, below are some ideas for how you can support your surrogate and her family.

Food deliveries and meal preparation. This is an obvious one, but may require more thinking to get it right. Find out what meals your surrogate and her family will eat – perhaps ask her or her partner to write a list of four or five meals that they know they will eat, and even steal their favourite recipes to make them. Fussy kids are unlikely to eat your gourmet degustation menu, so focus on practical and healthy foods that are easy to freeze and reheat. If you live far away from your surrogate, you might like to arrange a road trip to fill their freezer with food. You might also consider meal delivery services, or vouchers for the local take-away shop. Running errands and doing the grocery shop is a great way to be helpful and take some pressure off the surrogate's family. If you are on the way to shops, check in with them and see what they need, that you can collect on your way.

Do not ask her, 'Can I help?' or say, 'Let me know if you need anything.' Her answer will almost always be 'No, thanks.' Surrogates are proud and they do not like feeling needy or relying on others to help. Instead, try 'I will be cooking for you, so let me know what meals you would like,' or 'I will come over and care for your kids while you have a massage; let me know what day suits.' Give her the massage voucher as well and she will feel better about accepting the help.

Hiring a cleaner, particularly when your surrogate is heavily pregnant or unwell, will alleviate some pressure in their home. Doing the dishes at 36 weeks pregnant is no one's idea of fun, and vacuuming and gardening can lead to killer back pain. You can contribute to the housework as well, but sometimes outsourcing makes it easier for everyone.

Babysitting the surrogate's children and letting her and her partner go out on a date night is a great way to offer support. Often, the relationship between the surrogate and her partner is the least of everyone's priorities (after pregnancy appointments, kids, housework, work...) and it is a crucial relationship to support. If you spend time with their children, you are giving them respite to spend time together. You are also building relationships with the children, which is important too.

Give your surrogate and her family space. This might seem counter-intuitive – after all, should you not be supportive all the time? Pregnancy is full-time, but much of it is boring and there is no reason why you need to be in each other's pockets all the time. Follow her lead, ask her for her input, but do not smother her with attention.

Help out with life admin. If your surrogate has a lot on her plate, offer to make appointments for the surrogacy and pregnancy. Help her complete paperwork and give her checklists of things she has to do. The administrative stuff involved in surrogacy can be boring and overwhelming – you can help by project-managing much of it, and leaving her to do the things she needs to do. You might like to have a shared documents folder where everyone in the team can keep up with the paperwork, and a shared calendar for appointments.

Help with home maintenance if you can. You may not need to plunge her toilet when it is blocked, but there is no harm in taking out the bins, sweeping the patio, mowing the lawn and alleviating the pressure on their household. If she has a cat, it is now your job to empty the kitty litter when you visit too.

Spend time with her. Did I mention this is one of my love languages? Surrogates do not want to spend all their time with you talking about surrogacy and pregnancy. Spend time with her talking about and doing other things. Take her out for lunch or bring her lunch, watch a movie together, attend the school fete together, spend time together as families. She will appreciate that the relationships are as important to you as they are to her and her family.

Another easy way to support your surrogate and her family: vouchers. Massage vouchers, book vouchers, movie vouchers, ten-pin bowling vouchers – activities and ways for her and her family to wind down and not worry about money.

Care packages for your surrogate. Care packages, at any time or at milestones, can be a lovely way to show appreciation.

You should speak to her partner or do some discrete investigative work to find out what she likes and where her interests lie. Here are a few suggestions.

- Chocolate and sweet treats
- Heat bag
- Medicines and herbal remedies for symptoms of the IVF drugs or pregnancy
- Hand creams and body lotions
- Massage vouchers, a spa voucher, pedicure or manicure (or all of them!)
- Books
- Herbal teas
- Pyjamas – get the size right!
- Flowers
- Candles

The surrogate's partner's needs

The intended parents should treat the surrogate and her partner as equal members of the team, and ensure they have built the relationship and trust with both of them. The partner needs to feel appreciated for the time and energy they put into surrogacy too. Partners may also have trouble asking for help, so sometimes the intended parents need to be creative in how they provide support.

Overall, the surrogate team and the intended parents need to remember that the surrogate's partner is as much a part of the process and the team as the surrogate. Without her partner's support, she is unlikely to be able to proceed with the surrogacy. The partner's investment and commitment to the arrangement is crucial. And not simply for a good journey, but for the relationships that grow out of surrogacy – the partner's relationship with the intended parents will be lifelong, and is worth investing in.

Kids and surrogacy

I'm often asked about my children's responses to me being a surrogate, and for advice about preparing children for surrogacy. My kids were taught fairly early that sperm + egg + uterus = baby. They are still learning about heterosexual sex being one way to make a baby, but in the beginning we simply explained it in terms that they could grasp. We explained that our first son Archie was conceived through IVF, because Mummy and Daddy needed help to make a baby and the doctor gave us that help. Archie likes that story; I think it makes him feel special that we went to so much effort to create him.

We started talking about me being a surrogate when Archie,

who was six at the time, asked about his friend who had two mums – why did his friend not have a dad? We talked about some kids having a mum and a dad, or two mums, or two dads. He knew that I had been an egg donor, that some of his friends were conceived with the help of a donor, and that at the time, our friend was pregnant with a child conceived with one of my eggs. He was surprised that two men could have a baby; he laughed and said, 'But how? They do not have a uterus!' I explained that sometimes a woman like me would carry the baby in my uterus, and that the baby would have two dads. Archie was satisfied with this explanation, perhaps because donor conception was already familiar to him.

As the time drew closer for me to start trying to conceive a child for our intended parents, we talked in more specific terms about our friends wanting a baby, and that Mummy would carry the baby for them. We talked about the baby growing in my belly, but that the baby would go home with our friends, and not home with us. Both my children – by this time aged about seven and four – wanted to know if we would see the baby, and could they cuddle the baby? Of course! We could visit and the baby would visit us.

I am often asked how my children coped with the surrogacy pregnancy and the baby not coming home with us. Remember that we only know what we know, and my kids did not know any different than what we told them. They knew that the baby was not coming home with us – there was no grief about this; it was just matter-of-fact. We talked about the pregnancy and what was happening to my body, and why Mummy could not bend down to pick up their toys. Some of the biggest discussions in our household were about the birth plans and arrangements for someone to care for our kids while I was at the hospital. We made sure the kids understood what to expect if they woke up to find a babysitter in the house, and that they would be able to visit me and the baby in hospital when the time was right.

When I gave birth and was away in hospital for a few days, our kids were excited for news updates and to be able to come and visit us in the hospital. Shortly after we left the hospital, we visited our intended parents and the baby in their home. We explained that I might be a bit sore and maybe even a bit teary in the first few weeks, and that they could ask questions but there was nothing to worry about – Mummy was happy that the baby was here and with her dads. But giving birth was tiring and I needed lots of rest and hugs. Our son Raf, who was almost five when the baby was born, drew a picture of all of us, and it was lovely to see him excited about our new family. Both kids took photographs of themselves with the baby to show their friends at school.

Since then, the kids have an understanding that there are some women who are surrogates like Mummy, but our surrogacy journey does not rate a mention. They look forward to spending time with our intended parents and the baby, and they dote on her the way they dote on their baby cousin. Sometimes babies are fun, but sometimes Lego is more interesting.

My advice for anyone needing to explain surrogacy to children is to be honest and keep it simple. There are plenty of books available that can help tell the story of donor conception and surrogacy. Remember, kids do not need complex, scientific explanations for something that is, ultimately, a story of love:

that the intended parents would like a baby, and the surrogate is going to help them have one. Involve them in the story, answer their questions honestly and give them the language to understand and be able to explain it to other people. It's not that complicated.

The baby shower

Celebrations and family parties take on a new dimension when a surrogacy arrangement facilitates the growing of a family. While the intended parents may be excited and proud to celebrate their impending arrival, as with so many things with surrogacy, the situation may be more complicated than it first appears. The baby shower is a celebration of the baby in the surrogate's belly. It cannot be separated from her, and therefore the celebration needs to involve and acknowledge her too. Remember, she does not want the spotlight – most surrogates feel uncomfortable with people (many of whom might be strangers) staring at her. It can also feel dissociating to be pregnant with someone else's child so, while she wants acknowledgement that she is doing a wonderful thing, she does not want to be objectified. Discussing the event with her and including her in the event are vital steps to celebrating this event in an inclusive manner.

CHAPTER 11

Birth

Birth options

We talked already about private and public healthcare for surrogacy pregnancies in the last chapter. As most surrogates will have birthed their own children before becoming a surrogate, they will have their own pregnancy and birth history, and ideas and intentions for how they imagine the surrogacy birth.

Some surrogates have particular needs and expectations about the surrogacy birth, based on how they birthed their own children. This might, for example, include repeat caesarean section, a vaginal birth after caesarean (VBAC), or a homebirth. Their birth history might include birthing after 40 weeks, or birthing before 38 weeks, and these factors might impact on their pregnancy and birth, and how their pregnancy is supported by their healthcare provider.

There are no rules or laws that dictate how a surrogacy birth must be managed. It is an individual discussion between the team and their healthcare provider, and what is best for the surrogate and the baby. Each pregnancy is different, and in the case of surrogacy the genetics of the baby will impact on the pregnancy and the baby's size and health.

As there are no laws dictating a surrogacy pregnancy or birth care, there are no reasons why a surrogate cannot make decisions about the sort of birth she wants. Certainly, medical advice provided will impact on the decision but the fact that it is surrogacy does not of itself determine the way, or when, the baby will be born.

A note about homebirth and hospital birth. Some surrogates have a preference for one or the other. Birth options and plans should be discussed between the parties early on in the journey. If there are deal-breakers on these topics, they should be discussed and negotiated before going any further. Surrogates want the best possible birth for themselves and the baby; it is important that intended parents release some control over the situation and decide whether they can support a surrogate regardless of her birth choices.

Birth planning

Intended parents and surrogates might think the birth is a simple matter of a baby being born and handed to the intended parents. When considered in more detail, there are some complex issues that need discussing amongst the team. Below are some discussion points for the team to consider when planning a surrogacy birth. You may access a free template birth plan via my website (see Additional resources on page 166). While some sceptics bemoan the use of a birth plan, setting intentions for the birth can help to clarify everyone's positions and expectations which hopefully reduces any misunderstandings, trauma and stress. Some of these topics will be subject to negotiation and advocacy with the healthcare provider and hospital.

1. **Who will attend the birth?**
   Both intended parents, or just one? Will the surrogate's partner be there?
2. **Support people**
   Will the surrogate have a support person, in addition or instead of her partner? Will she have a doula or private midwife in attendance?
3. **Birth photographer**
4. **Childcare arrangements**
   Who will care for the children during the labour and birth?
5. **Pain relief**
6. **Catching the baby**
7. **Cord clamping and cutting the cord**
8. **First cuddles and skin-to-skin contact**
9. **Discovering and announcing the baby's sex (if not already known)**
10. **Who will stay with the baby and who will stay with the surrogate if they need to be separated?**
11. **Milk and feeding**
12. **Placenta delivery and use**
13. **Contact between the parties while in hospital**
14. **Room arrangements**
15. **Leaving the hospital**
16. **Announcing the birth**

Hospital management

There are low number of surrogacy births in Australia each year, and it is no surprise that many hospitals will rarely come across a surrogacy birth. As a result, hospital surrogacy policies can be outdated or inflexible, and not apply to a surrogacy arrangement the way the parties hoped.

For example, some hospital surrogacy policies will declare that only the birth mother can feed the baby, and not the intended parents. They may also refuse to allow the intended parents to remain in hospital with the baby, pressuring them to depart after visiting hours and leave the baby in the birth mother's care.

At the back of this book you will find a drafted 'Best practice guidelines for care in surrogacy', which hospitals and care providers can use to write their own surrogacy policy.

The hospital may have their lawyers review the surrogacy agreement and birth plan and advise whether the intended parents can care for the baby and leave the hospital with the baby separately to the birth mother. Sometimes, the hospital will request a document with the birth parents' consent to the intended parents caring for and leaving hospital with the baby. A parenting plan can meet this need if necessary.

If you are facing hurdles with your chosen care providers, request a meeting with the relevant staff (such as the nurse unit manager or hospital social worker).

Continuity of care

Ask if the hospital is able to provide the team with one primary point of contact to assist in continuity of care and support.

Continuity of care is proven to improve birth outcomes and experiences.

Ideally, the surrogate should have one-to-one care during the pregnancy. This might not be possible, but it is an important consideration. Surrogates and intended parents do not want to have to re-tell their story to a new midwife or doctor at every appointment.

Birth education and parent craft for the intended parents

Ask if the hospital will provide 'parent craft' and birth education for the intended parents. The birth and parent craft classes are usually offered to pregnant people and their partners, but your surrogate may not want or need to attend. If you are not comfortable attending a hospital birth class as intended parents, you might like to have private birth classes with a midwife. Some private birth workers understand the complexity of surrogacy arrangements, and others will be LGBTQI+ friendly.

Intended parents in the birthing suite or theatre

Will the intended parents be welcomed into the birthing suite, or theatre, should there be a caesarean birth? Most hospitals will have policies that the birthing person can only have one support person with them in theatre. You should ask the hospital to reconsider this policy for your team, so that both intended parents can see the birth of their baby if the surrogate wishes. Hopefully, the surrogate's partner would also be allowed in theatre. Some teams have been successful in having a birth photographer in theatre or recovery.

A room for the intended parents

After a surrogacy birth, the surrogate will hopefully be able to recover and be attended in her own room, and the intended parents will get to know their new baby in a separate room nearby. However, public hospitals might not have the room and private hospitals may charge the intended parents to stay in a separate room. You need to discuss this with the hospital. Sometimes, the surrogate and one of the intended parents will share a room with the baby, if no separate room can be provided. The surrogate should not be made to care for the baby while the intended parents go home at the end of visiting hours. The hospital will need to be educated about the inappropriateness of such an arrangement and the potentially harmful impact on everyone involved.

Milk and feeding

Some intended mothers will want to induce lactation, and you should mention this to the hospital prior to the birth. I have heard of hospitals refusing to allow the intended mother to breastfeed her own baby because they consider that only the legal parent (the surrogate) is allowed to care or feed the baby. You should avoid the stress of it becoming a problem by speaking to the hospital well in advance and gaining their support. (See later in this chapter for more on milk and feeding.)

Birth photography

Birth photography is an art form. You only need to search #birth-photo on social media and find out how popular and amazing it can be.

Many teams will consider that birth photography is a nice, indulgent idea, but not necessary. And considering the amount of money the intended parents will have spent by the time the birth happens, it is understandable that they might not want to spend more money on a non-essential thing like photography.

However, in my opinion, birth photography is an essential part a surrogacy birth. The key moment for the surrogate is when she sees the intended parents meet their baby for the first time. This might be in the birthing suite, or theatre, or in recovery. When that moment is compromised – perhaps by pain medication, or someone standing between the surrogate and the intended parents, or by an emergency in the birthing room – the surrogate can lose or forget that moment. And this is not a moment she can repeat. If that moment is not captured, the surrogate can spend a lot of time trying to process the birth and those crucial first moments. If the birth became an emergency, or was traumatic, her trauma may be magnified by the fact that she did not see the intended parents meet the baby she carried for nine months.

Birth photographers can bridge that gap. And not just for the surrogate, but for the intended parents, and the surrogate's partner and support people as well. And for the child, when they are older, it can provide them with vital images of their birth story.

Surrogates will picture the moment of the surrogacy birth in their minds for the entire pregnancy, and often before a pregnancy is achieved. They imagine what it will be like, who will be there, and will play out the moment that the intended parents see their baby for the first time in their mind, over and over.

It is important to find a birth photographer who understands surrogacy, or who is open to learning about it. They should be willing to learn about the dynamics in your team and understand how you imagine the birth. They need to understand why images of the birth are important to the team, and particularly to the surrogate. You might consider nominating someone within your team to take photos, but the reality is that everyone will be (and should be) entirely absorbed in what is happening, not taking photos of it. You want everyone to be in the photos, and not taking blurry photos in bad lighting. You have one chance at getting it right, and my advice would be to pay a professional to do it for you.

If you are considering hiring a birth photographer, there is a lot to think about. To help you make the right decision for your team, consider these points.

- Talk about it with your team: set birth photography as an agenda item and decide if it's important to your team.
- Reach agreements about sharing the photos. You might have an agreement about which photos to share and with whom. Will the birth video be uploaded to YouTube? Or only seen by the team?
- If you are not hiring a professional photographer, consider nominating a team member to take photos. Perhaps the surrogate's partner or support person?
- Make sure the photographer knows to capture the moment of birth and everyone's reactions. This might

mean trying to capture two things at the same time! This is really important – the surrogate wants to see everyone's faces as they meet their baby!

- If you are hiring a professional photographer, give them a brief about who is in your team, and talk to them about how surrogacy works and why photography is important to you. Meet them beforehand and find out if they are a good match for you.
- Another benefit of birth photography is that it normalises birth. Intended parents who have not birthed or observed birth before might find it useful to watch YouTube videos of birth and look at birth photographs on social media. Our birth photos have started many a conversation, and hopefully helped to de-stigmatise surrogacy and educate people about the beauty of birth, surrogacy, and the family we created.

Handing over the baby

Feelings at birth

One of the many questions that surrogates will ask other surrogates when considering their future birth is whether they will cope with handing over the baby, or whether their hormones will overcome their rational brain. 'Will I lose my head? Will I have a meltdown?' The good news is that mostly, surrogates report having a positive experience during the post-partum period. For many of us, the overwhelming feelings are that of love and joy and positive feelings about handing the baby to their parents. But mixed with those feelings are good dose of hormones and confusion about how we are meant to feel. When I gave birth, I felt overwhelmed with positive feelings – but that was also confusing. I wondered whether there was a guide book for how I was meant to feel, and where I was meant to channel the overwhelming joy that I felt. There were very few people I could talk to about this, because the only people with a similar experience were other surrogates. Many surrogates report feeling that they cannot talk about their feelings with their friends or family because everyone is expecting that they will fall apart at any moment. There is an expectation in society that giving away a baby must be traumatic, so expressing anything other than joy is risky for a surrogate wanting to explore the complex emotions she is feeling.

Debunking fears around handing over the baby

One of the first questions asked by intended parents considering surrogacy in Australia is 'What if she wants to keep the baby?'

And one of the first questions asked by a surrogate and her partner is 'What if they do not take the baby?'

You may laugh at the irony of those two questions, and certainly many surrogates will scoff at the idea that they will want to keep the baby. If an intended parent is anxious about the prospect of their surrogate refusing to hand over the baby, there is not much that can give them 100 per cent certainty that it will not happen.

So here are some facts that might help. And while they are meant to help, they are in no way meant to diminish an intended parent's understandable concerns.

Most surrogates can conceive and carry a baby with their

partner without medical or legal intervention, let alone blood tests, invasive physical examinations, police checks, counselling or involving another couple in their family planning. They do not want to have any baby; they want to have your baby and give it to you. This might seem a strange idea – why would anyone want to have a baby for someone else? Everything in altruistic surrogacy comes back to the intentions of everyone involved. If the baby was conceived with the intention that it is to be raised and loved by the intended parents, it would feel very strange for the surrogate to consider raising the baby herself. In fact, it could feel like grief. As surrogates, we become entirely invested in you becoming parents. If that expectation is not fulfilled, we can grieve for it. The idea that we would keep a baby we never intended keeping feels absurd. And this applies to traditional and gestational surrogates – even if we have a genetic connection to the baby, we never intended bringing it home. The baby is yours – you can have it.

Yes, your baby is gorgeous and delightful and goodness that newborn smell is intoxicating! And still, we do not want to take it home with us. Some of us are even willing to breast-feed and have skin-to-skin contact with the baby after the birth – and hand it over without any problems. Hormones are amazing, pregnancy and birth is amazing. Still, we do not want your baby. Our body might react to the baby's presence, and so it should – we carried the baby for nine months, it would be strange if we did not respond. But here is the thing: the human brain is complex, and humans are capable of complex feelings and thoughts. I can simultaneously love my children and enjoy the time they are in school. Likewise, we can love your baby and have a physical reaction to baby, and still not want to raise it and take it home with us. Actually, we would rather see you doing all the parenting, because that is what we always intended.

Most people have an idea of what their family will look like. It changes over time, of course. Intended parents will understand the desire to have children is partly to do with how you see your future, and your expectations of raising children and when that might happen. Likewise, surrogates also have ideas about what their family looks like. For me, I was adamant that two kids was right for us. We considered adding a third, but it didn't feel right. Our car fits two kids comfortably, we can holiday with two kids easily, we have goals that include two kids – and not three, or four. So, imagine if that image of family changes because another child arrives, unexpectedly. For me, the idea of a third child was out of the question. The possibility of having to raise surro-baby in our family was terrifying, and this possibility often causes anxiety for surrogates and their partners. I remember cuddles with newborn surro-baby made me anxious – I hadn't planned on looking after a newborn! Why did they keep handing her to me?!

'But what about the law?' I hear you ask. You are right: Australian laws provide that surrogacy arrangements are not enforceable. At birth, the surrogate and her partner are the baby's legal parents – for a bit, anyway. If the surrogate decides to keep the baby, by law there is nothing the intended parents can do to enforce the surrogacy agreement. They can go to the family courts, where the decision of where the baby lives would be about the baby's best interests, not based on the surrogacy agreement.

Why is this? Well, because you cannot have a contract on a baby (that's akin to child trafficking), and you cannot have a contract on a woman's body. These are two fundamental legal principles that are maintained and are unlikely to change any time soon. But the statistics for a surrogate keeping the baby in Australia since decent surrogacy laws were introduced (10 years ago in most states) are 0 per cent. Nil. Zero. Certainly, there have been some negative outcomes where the surrogate and intended parents have not been friends after the birth . . . and still, the surrogate has not tried to keep the baby.

In commercial surrogacy arrangements in the US, the chances of the surrogate keeping the baby are five times less likely than the intended parents refusing to take the baby. Think that over for a moment. Intended parents are more likely to refuse to take the baby than a surrogate is likely to want to keep it. So, who takes the biggest risk?

How does it feel to give away a baby?

Probably the most common question I have received since I gave birth is 'How does it feel, to give a baby away?' And usually the follow up comment is 'I could never give away a baby.' Do not worry. I thought that too, once a upon a time. I think surrogates appreciate that giving away a baby is pretty weird to most people, unless they really understand surrogacy. But while it might seem weird and even outrageous, it is important to remember that on the whole, surrogates are well-adjusted, well-supported and happy to be doing what they're doing. The worst response you can give them is sympathy – I had people say, 'Oh that must have been so hard.' Trust me when I say that while surrogacy is complex, giving a baby to the intended parents is not the hard part.

The short answer is: it was amazing. It was one of the best things I have ever done in my entire life. Not once have I ever regretted any of it. It is the gift that keeps giving back – every time I see her with her dads, I feel a rush of love and pride and joy that I played a part in her being here. I get to experience that for the rest of my life.

The long answer is a little more complex. Babies born through surrogacy are conceived with the intention that they will be raised by the intended parents, not by the birth parents. At every moment, well before the conception takes place, the birth mother thinks she will be handing over the baby. She thinks about that moment a lot. She is excited for the moment that she can see the intended parents with their baby.

When it comes to handing over the baby to the intended parents, it is not just something we are happy to do, it is something that feels completely natural and wonderful, and we do not have a second thought about it. I have not met a surrogate who has reconsidered whether she would hand over the baby at the birth.

The team will have their own surrogacy birth plan and ideas for what happens at the birth and in the days afterwards. And while birth sometimes does not go according to plan, the surrogate handing over the baby and the intended parents taking care of the baby is pretty straightforward. The intended parents will return home with the baby, and the surrogate will return home to her family.

There is something that I think we can take away from

surrogacy as part of the human experience. Society has very clear ideas of what motherhood should be like, and how mothers should behave. We are expected to enjoy every second of motherhood, and feel absolutely devoted and connected to our children 100 per cent of the time. I think surrogacy challenges this idea – I gave birth to a baby, genetically related to me, and I gave her to someone else to raise, and did not grieve for her. There is scientific research that shows that what we might consider 'maternal instinct' is in fact an increase in oxytocin, which anyone can experience even if they have not birthed the baby. It was indeed what I observed – my intended parents responded to the baby the way I responded to my two children when they were born. I did not respond to the baby in the same way. I likened it to how I might respond if my friends had a baby. I love the baby, I think she is amazing, but I did not feel any 'instinct' to care for her or respond to her needs. The idea that I might have to care for her was, frankly, terrifying.

It can also seem rather reductive to suggest that a surrogate must grieve when she hands over a baby that was intended for other people to raise. It says that women are slaves to our hormones and our 'motherly instinct', and that we are simple creatures not capable of complex emotions – like loving a child and not wanting to care for it. The more I learn about surrogacy and motherhood, the more I know that humans are complex and capable of a range of thoughts and emotions.

Does the surrogate have legal rights at birth?

Given that surrogacy agreements in Australia are not enforceable, many intended parents will wonder whether a surrogate has legal rights or parentage when the baby is born, and before or after a parentage order is granted.

At the time of the birth, the surrogate and her partner are the legal parents. In practice, and what you can expect in the post-partum period, is that the surrogate will relinquish the child to the intended parents at the birth, and she will do none of the newborn care or parenting. The intended parents perform all those tasks, and the team can have any agreements they wish as to who cuts the cord at birth, how baby is fed and who has the first cuddle. You can read more about milk and feeding the baby below.

The intended parents can perform all the parenting tasks expected of new parents, including taking baby home with them and staying up all night watching their newborn's facial expressions. The surrogate and her partner will return home and settle back into their usual routine without needing to be involved in any of the baby's care. So while the surrogate and her partner are technically the legal parents, in practice their involvement is minimal.

If the baby requires medical treatment prior to the parentage order being made, the surrogate and her partner may be required to sign consent forms for this to occur. If the intended parents take the baby to a doctor the Medicare card will likely suffice to obtain treatment.

Once the parentage order is granted, parentage is transferred from the birth parents to the intended parents (see chapter 14 for more information about parentage orders). At that time, the intended parents have full parental responsibility in the legal sense and will be listed on a new birth certificate. The birth parents will have no legal responsibility for the baby, and any future relationship between the birth parents and the baby is determined by the intended parents and what is considered in the child's best interests.

What happens legally if the birth parents choose not to relinquish the child to the intended parents?

When we say that surrogacy agreements are not enforceable, what we are really saying is that they are not binding in the Family Court. No agreement about children made between parents or other people binds the court unless it is made into an order of the court. In the case where the birth parents decide not to relinquish the child to the intended parents, they remain the legal parents but this does not necessarily mean that they will be granted parental responsibility for the child. If the intended parents make an application to the Family Court to have the child placed in their care, the court will consider all the evidence and primarily what is in the child's best interests. This means that the decision of who cares for and raises the child is up to the court, not to the birth parents or the intended parents. And while this might seem worrying for anyone entering into a surrogacy arrangement, this is entirely how it should be if we are to maintain that the child's interests are paramount, and not the interests of either the birth parents or the intended parents.

Milk and feeding

All new parents must grapple with learning how to feed their newborn and making the right decisions for the family. When you add in surrogacy, it can take on a whole other level of complexity. Be reassured, there is no wrong or right answer – formula or breastmilk, induced lactation, or a combination of the three. What is right for you and your team and family may not be right for everyone.

While I am a strong advocate for fed is best, there are many benefits for the baby and the surrogate for her to provide colostrum (the first milk produced and ideal nourishment for a newborn) and breastmilk for the baby, for any length of time.

When making a decision about what is right for you and your team, there are many options to consider. Some options for feeding the new baby in a surrogacy arrangement might include the following.

The surrogate expresses colostrum leading up to the birth so that there is a stock of milk ready for when the baby is born. Some surrogates have managed to express enough colostrum to satisfy a hungry newborn for the first 24 hours or longer.

The surrogate might continue to express breastmilk for the intended parents to feed the baby for several weeks or months after the birth. Some surrogates find expressing difficult and stop, while others continue for several months and have a large supply. The decision to express might also be impacted by whether the intended parents live nearby or if the milk needs to travel to them.

The surrogate might direct breastfeed in the hours or days after the birth. For some surrogates, this is the easiest way to get colostrum to the baby and is also a lovely way to connect with the baby after the birth. Direct feeding and/or skin to skin between surrogate and baby is an important part of the fourth stage of labour, when the body recognises that the birth is over and the baby has arrived and is safe.

Many surrogates will not express colostrum or breastmilk, in which case the baby usually goes straight on formula from the birth. The intended parents may consider sourcing donated breastmilk from Human Milk 4 Human Babies and other sources.

Intended mothers might consider inducing lactation so they can breastfeed the baby themselves. Induced lactation is a long process and requires assistance from medication and a supportive GP. It is worth researching further if you are interested. There are many intended mothers who have induced lactation and successfully breastfed the baby upon their arrival. If you are interested, start a conversation with your GP and seek the support and information from other women who have successfully induced lactation. There are online support groups available, in addition to medical treatment.

The decision as to how the baby will be fed should be made as a team, with open minds and having considered the options.

There are many reasons why a surrogate might provide milk for the baby if she wants to, which benefit her and the baby. Likewise, there are many reasons why some surrogates would prefer not to feed or provide milk for the baby. If you are an intended parent and are uncomfortable with the idea of your surrogate feeding the baby, you should talk it through with your team and consider whether you can overcome the discomfort or not.

Rest assured, a surrogate who breastfeeds and has skin-to-skin contact with the baby will not become too attached to the baby, and this will not affect her ability to hand the baby over. On the contrary, in my experience the breastfeeding of surrobaby felt as natural as handing her over to her fathers, and felt like a lovely long goodbye between her and I. My advice about breastmilk and feeding is to be flexible. Most teams are still adjusting their birth and feeding plans in the days leading up to and after the birth. Open communication and sensitivity should be the priority for everyone.

Announcing the birth

Have agreements about when and how the birth will be announced. Once it is announced, everyone will be inundated with messages and this can take away from the energy you should be spending on each other. If you are announcing the birth to anyone – whether privately or on social media – you should include your surrogate and acknowledge her and her family. She may not want to be tagged in a Facebook post, but unless your friends think a stork brought you a baby, include her name in the announcement.

Be prepared for unwelcome gawkers

Be prepared to set clear boundaries with outsiders who may wish to rubber-neck and gossip about the surrogacy. While the intended parent's families and friends will be celebrating the new baby, the surrogate may be dealing with intrusive questions about how she is coping and whether she is falling apart. You may need to limit contact with anyone who is not part of the immediate support circle. Remember that the surrogate, her partner and the intended parents have been through an enormous and life-changing event; not everyone needs to gawk at the aftermath.

Leaving the hospital

The team should consider the logistics of the surrogate and baby leaving the hospital together or separately. If either needs to remain in hospital while the other is ready to leave, the hospital should accommodate that. However, this is often cause for problems as the hospital considers the surrogate is the legal mother at that time, and may not be willing to allow the baby to leave without her. The team should discuss with the hospital staff, management, or the social worker what the hospital needs to allow the baby to leave without the surrogate. Some teams have provided the hospital with a parenting plan, which is a written document signed by the birth parents, relinquishing the baby to the intended parents. It is not binding, but can satisfy the hospital that the baby is in safe hands leaving with the intended parents.

Returning home with baby from overseas

Intended parents engaging in overseas surrogacy are anxious to make sure they can bring their baby home without falling foul of overseas or Australian laws, or being stuck at a border and unable to come home. Make sure to get advice about your specific circumstances, and from a wide range of sources. You should consult a lawyer in your destination country, ensuring that they have experience with Australian intended parents and will assist you to leave their country with your baby. You should also discuss your particular arrangement and circumstances with an Australian lawyer and a migration agent.

When your baby is born, there are a raft of processes and bureaucracy that you need to get your baby out of the country and into Australia. Much of the information you need is available from the Home Affairs website, which is an Australian government website with information about passports, visas, returning to Australia with your baby, and Citizenship by Descent.

Pre- or post-birth order

The legal documents to recognise you as the parent/s of the child are arranged by the agency and lawyer in your destination country. The lawyer should advise you about this process and undertake all necessary work involved. You should not need an Australian lawyer to facilitate this process.

Obtaining a passport from the country of birth

Most intended parents obtain a passport for their baby from the destination country, and then bring baby to Australia on a temporary visa. However, some countries consider the child 'stateless' and will not issue a passport for the child. In that case, you will be applying for Australian Citizenship by Descent first, and an Australian passport to bring baby to Australia.

Obtaining a visa for the baby to travel to Australia

You can either apply for a visa to bring your baby into Australia or apply for Citizenship by Descent. Do not do them simultaneously as one cancels out the other. If you are arriving in Australia with your baby on a temporary visa, you can apply for Citizenship by Descent upon arrival.

Returning to Australia

Other parents who have travelled with newborns are a wealth of information. Contact the airline and ask for seats next to a bassinet. Find out about travelling with liquids and pre-prepared formula. Carry all documents with you, including the birth certificate, passports, visa documentation, Citizenship by Descent (if applicable) and the surrogacy contract.

Citizenship by Descent

You can apply for Citizenship by Descent if your baby was born outside Australia and either of the parents is an Australian citizen. You can apply for Citizenship by Descent online, after the birth and before you arrive home, or when you arrive back in Australia. Citizenship by Descent requires evidence that the child is your descendant, either by genetics or intention. You may also be required to provide a copy of the surrogacy and donor agreements and the birth certificate. The best source of information for the Citizenship by Descent application is at the Home Affairs website: immi.homeaffairs.gov.au.

Medicare and Centrelink for babies born overseas

Your child is eligible for Medicare rebates and medical treatment under Medicare even if they were born overseas. If a child enters Australia on a foreign passport, they can access Medicare if they are Australian citizens and have come to live in Australia. They will become eligible once their citizenship is established.

Do we need parentage orders or parenting orders if we are coming home from overseas?

Intended parents entering into commercial surrogacy arrangements overseas are often anxious to know about returning home to Australia with their baby, any consequences, and whether they need to get court orders when they return to Australia.

Parentage orders are made to transfer parentage from a surrogate and her partner to the intended parents. These are made in state courts. These orders provide for the birth certificate to be changed, removing the surrogate and her partner, and replacing their names with those of the intended parents. Parentage orders granted in this form are only available for surrogacy arrangements entered into in Australia (see chapter 14 for more information).

Parenting orders are often made when parents are separated and need to formalise the arrangements for where the children will live and who they will spend time with. These are made in the Family Court.

In some international surrogacy cases, intended parents have chosen to obtain parenting orders to recognise both parents as having parental responsibility for the child, once they return to Australia. This is generally not necessary where both the intended parents are already listed on the birth certificate, unless they are separating.

You may be told that you must have a parenting order if you had a child through international surrogacy. This is usually not the case. Parenting orders can only be obtained if you have evidence of the surrogacy arrangement and can provide evidence that the surrogate and her partner consented to the order being made. The parenting order application process can be complex, time-consuming and expensive – if you do not need to do it, why would you bother? If only one (or neither) of the intended parents is listed on the birth certificate, parenting orders can provide acknowledgment that the intended parents have parental responsibility of the child (and that the surrogate does not), and can assist with accessing services such as Medicare and Centrelink.

Much has been written about Australian family laws and recognising parentage of children born through overseas surrogacy. Many parents return from overseas and do not need a court order or to register an overseas order to behave like parents, obtain Citizenship by Descent and an Australian passport, access services and enrol their child in childcare and school.

The legal process to apply for the order is expensive and very often, no order is granted. My short advice is: do not fix it if it is not broken. Spend your money on your new baby, not more lawyers. If you do strike trouble with any of those things after you return to Australia, you can contact a lawyer to discuss your options.

CHAPTER 12

The fourth trimester

Many people will not have heard of the fourth trimester, let alone when it applies in a surrogacy arrangement. The fourth trimester refers to the first three months after a baby is born when the baby is going through a period of massive growth and change and getting used to the outside world. It also refers to the period of the parents growing into their new roles. And in surrogacy, it refers to the surrogate's period of getting used to no longer being pregnant, her new role in the intended parents' and baby's lives, and adjusting to life beyond surrogacy. It is arguably the most challenging and amazing part of the entire surrogacy. It is important to respect the fourth trimester as a period of great change for everyone, a time which demands respect and gentleness with ourselves and each other, and a time of transition from being part of a surrogacy arrangement to lifelong friends.

The surrogate has to manage the hormonal and physical changes as well as adjusting to life beyond surrogacy. Her head knows that the baby is where she intended and is loved and cared for with the intended parents. Her body needs time to catch up and adjust to that reality. The biggest change in hormones occurs in the days and weeks after a woman gives birth. The surrogate may find herself confused – as I did – that her body looks like that of a postnatal woman, as if she has forgotten the recent birth and the baby. Some surrogates report seeing the baby with the intended parents and having to remind themselves that they birthed the baby. The fourth trimester can feel like an emotional rollercoaster, even when it goes well.

Surrogates and intended parents can prepare for a smooth and happy fourth trimester, and it will be different for everyone. Surrogates have to adjust back to life as a mother and partner, no longer being pregnant without having a baby in her arms, and no longer being a surrogate. Some planning and flexibility are advisable for everyone, and care for each other and self is crucial during this period of huge transition.

Debrief the birth

This is more important than most people realise and can be a crucial part of transitioning from surrogacy to the new normal. Even if the labour and birth went to plan, debriefing can help everyone process the enormous event of birth and your feelings about it. If the birth did not go as you had planned or hoped, it can help you process it so that it doesn't keep you awake at night. The surrogate might like to debrief the birth privately with a counsellor or midwife, but doing it together as a team can be really useful as well.

Fourth-trimester counselling

Counselling in the fourth trimester is a requirement for the parentage order application in most states. Many teams treat it like a tick-the-box process, but it can be helpful not only for debriefing the birth but also for adjusting and transitioning to the new normal post-surrogacy. Surrogates can benefit from speaking with a counsellor to help them clarify their feelings about their new role as the 'ex-surrogate' and give language to all their thoughts and feelings about the baby and the intended parents. Counselling, before during and after surrogacy, is not about crisis management or fixing something that is broken – it is a vital part of maintaining individual and team wellbeing and relationships.

Adjusting to life after being a surrogate

While the intended parents may be occupied with their newborn, getting back to normal life can take some time for a surrogate. Some things that might help with the transition for surrogates include the following.

Plan nice things to do

Make sure they are easy to arrange, flexible and nourishing. Have nice things planned that are good for the mind, good for the soul and good for the body.

Some nice things you might like:

1. Pedicure
2. Massage
3. A trip to an art gallery or museum

4. A brunch date with a friend
5. A picnic with your kids
6. Read a new book
7. A movie date with your partner.

Take it easy and be kind to yourself

Your body, hormones and mind might play tricks on you during the first few weeks. Many surrogates say that they forget that they have given birth or forget that the baby in the intended parents' arms is the baby they birthed. Your hormones might make you cry at the drop of a hat and you might not know why! And your body might be the only reminder that you just had a baby. I was shocked that my body looked like it had been recently pregnant because my mind was telling me to get on with my life. The biggest lesson here is that no two surrogates are the same, but we can probably relate to each other's experiences of the fourth trimester. Be kind to yourself – there is no rule book about how you will feel. Remind yourself that your body needs time to recover and you should not feel the need to get it back to its pre-pregnancy state too quickly.

A new project

Having a new project to keep you busy is one way to transfer the energies from the surrogacy to something else. It might be a craft project, or a new educational endeavour, or planning a family holiday. Be sure that the new project does not take too much physical or emotional energy or require too much brain power. You may find that you do not have the emotional or intellectual energy for anything too complex in the first few months.

Visits with surro-baby

Visits with your intended parents and the baby are a lovely way to see them as a family and bask in the glow of the surrogacy and what you did to help them become a family. If you are not able to see each other in person, FaceTime catchups and photos are almost as good. Many surrogates do not feel the need to see frequent updates from their intended parents, but being in close contact can be a lovely way to stay connected after the epic event of the birth and everything you have done together.

Post-birth care for the surrogate family

One thing that many teams do not plan for is what needs to happen if the surrogate and her family need assistance post-birth. This might be because she had a caesarean and cannot drive for six weeks. It might be because she has other post-birth complications and requires ongoing medical appointments. She is unlikely to be able to clean her house or return to work in the early weeks. Meanwhile, the intended parents are under-standably besotted and absorbed in their newborn. How is the team going to support each other and move through these early weeks to make sure the surrogate is getting the care and assis-tance she needs? Some things that might be needed include the following.

- A cleaner for the surrogate family
- Someone to assist with driving the surrogate family, or taxi vouchers
- Ready-made frozen meals for the surrogate family
- Open communication and regular contact between the team.

A perpetual journey

Surrogacy relationships are forever. Long after the baby is born and the parentage order is made, the team will be tied together for life. Much like a marriage, the relationship will sometimes be challenging but there is something keeping the parties together – the shared experience, and the child they created together. The first three months after the birth are the biggest and contain the most rapid changes in the relationship, but the changes continue long after the fourth trimester is officially over. It is a perpetual journey, with many periods of transition and adjustment before there is any sense of a new normal. My advice is to talk to other intended parents and surrogates, share your experience and find support in the community, and access counselling even before you think you need it. There is no wrong or right way to feel, and the chances are someone else has thought and felt very similarly to you. I have taken much wisdom and comfort from talking to other intended parents and surrogates, who understand and can relate to the experience.

CHAPTER 13

Registration and services

Birth registration

After the birth, it is the responsibility of all the parties to ensure that the baby's birth is registered. As the birth parents, the surrogate and her partner must be listed as the baby's parents on the original birth certificate.

The hospital will provide the surrogate and her partner with details about registering the baby's birth with the state Registry of Births, Deaths and Marriages.

The surrogate and her partner will be listed as the baby's parents.

The intended parents can choose the baby's first, middle and surnames. It is important that the child's name is a true reflection of the name that the parties intend for them to have for life. It is not appropriate to give the child the surrogate's surname unless you wish that to be permanent. If the child is registered with the wrong name, you will need to register a change of name before applying for a parentage order.

What if the surrogate is single?

The surrogate should list her details as the birth parent on the birth certificate. If she does not have a partner, she will need to provide details to the registry of the surrogacy arrangement. A copy of the surrogacy agreement should suffice. A letter from the IVF clinic may also be necessary to provide evidence of the conception.

What if the surrogate is in a same-sex female couple?

Both the surrogate and her partner should be listed as the birth parents on the birth certificate. As the registry will likely ask for details of the conception if the surrogate is in a same-sex female relationship, you will need to provide a copy of the surrogacy agreement when filing the birth registration.

Can the intended genetic father be listed on the original birth certificate?

Under Australian law, a woman who births a child is presumed to be the child's legal parent, and if she has a partner, they too are presumed to be a parent. In order to recognise the intended parents in a surrogacy arrangement, they must apply for a parentage order through their state court. In order to effect a transfer of parentage, the court needs to transfer parentage from the birth parents to the intended parents. If the intended father is listed on the birth certificate with the surrogate, then the court may have difficulty making a parentage order transferring parentage from the birth parents to the intended parents, and in those circumstances may declare that the original birth record must be amended before they will make a parentage order.

My advice is that the birth parents should always be listed on the original birth registration unless you have received specific legal advice to the contrary.

Birth certificates and overseas births

Both intended parents can be named on the birth certificate, regardless of any genetic link, in most destination countries. In some countries, the birth mother will be named on the birth certificate, or only one of the intended parents will be named. You should ask your lawyer in your destination country whether either or both intended parents will be named on the birth certificate and the process for this to occur.

Medicare

It is Medicare's practice to list a child on the Medicare card of the parents listed on the birth certificate. In surrogacy arrangements, this often results in the birth parents being mistakenly issued with a new Medicare card, listing the baby. This also means that the intended parents may need to jump extra hoops in order to access Medicare for the baby.

The team should try to visit a Medicare office together, in

person, and speak to a staff member about the surrogacy arrangement. You can take a copy of the surrogacy agreement with you and explain the situation. Medicare may issue a separate card for the child in their own name, until a parentage order is made.

If the child is listed on the birth parents' Medicare card, you may need to wait until the parentage order has been granted before rectifying the issue with Medicare.

Between the time of the birth and the parentage order being granted, the intended parents may need to take a photocopy or screenshot of the surrogate's Medicare card with them to any medical appointments for the baby.

Once the parentage order is granted, the intended parents can take a copy of the order with the new birth certificate listing them as parents, and seek that the Medicare record be updated and the child listed on their Medicare card.

If your baby was born overseas, you can apply for Medicare once you have arrived home and received the Citizenship by Descent.

Centrelink

Surrogates and intended parents can all apply for Centrelink's Paid Parental Leave Scheme (PPL). The surrogate can apply because she needs time to recover from the birth. The intended parents can apply as primary carer of the baby and partner of the primary carer.

Unfortunately, because surrogacy is not common in Australia, Centrelink staff may not be aware of their own policy and may determine that the surrogate cannot access PPL based on the baby not being in her care. However, Centrelink's own policy directs that the surrogate can apply for PPL, and most surrogates have been granted the benefit. My advice is that the birth parents should attend Centrelink with the intended parents to apply in person. If the staff are not familiar with the policy, then insist on speaking with someone who knows more about it. If you are refused the benefit and think you are eligible, then appeal the decision.

If your baby was born overseas, you can still apply for the PPL as the parent with the care of an infant child.

CHAPTER 14

The parentage order

Applying for a parentage order

After a baby is born in an Australian surrogacy arrangement, a parentage order is required to transfer parentage from the surrogate and her partner to the intended parents.

Once the birth certificate is issued, the intended parents must apply for a parentage order. They apply to a court in the state where they live. The purpose of a parentage order is to transfer parentage from the surrogate and her partner to the intended parents. This has the effect of providing an order that recognises the surrogacy arrangement, and who the true parents are. The order also tells the Registry of Births, Deaths and Marriages in the surrogate's state to re-issue the birth certificate with the parents listed, instead of the surrogate and her partner.

For the court to grant a parentage order, the intended parents will need to provide evidence of the surrogacy arrangement, and that the surrogate and her partner have relinquished care of the baby to the parents. This is usually provided by way of affidavits from each of the intended parents and the surrogate and her partner.

The court will need to see evidence that the parties received legal advice and counselling prior to the pregnancy. In most states, post-surrogacy counselling is also a requirement of the parentage order.

You should refer to the legislation in the state where the intended parents live to understand the requirements that apply to you.

Most intended parents engage a lawyer to assist them prepare the parentage order application. Some intended parents have been successful in preparing the application themselves. If you are wanting to be as ready as you can be for the application, you can collect some of the necessary documents, including:

- A signed and dated copy of the surrogacy agreement
- A copy of each of the legal advice letters or statements provided by the lawyers before everyone signed the agreement
- The counselling report from the pre-surrogacy counsellor
- If you needed a surrogate for medical reasons, you should have a letter from your treating doctor as to why you needed a surrogate. This might be from your fertility specialist
- The baby's birth certificate
- Certified copies of the intended parents' driver licences
- A letter from your IVF clinic confirming that they performed an embryo transfer and the date of the

transfer, and that it resulted in a pregnancy with the estimated due date

- The counselling report from the post-surrogacy counsellor.

Parentage order celebration

Parentage orders are made by the state courts, and each process is different. There might be a hearing that everyone can attend. In some states, parentage orders are made without a hearing and the judge will make the order 'in chambers.'

The parentage order marks an important milestone in the surrogacy journey. For intended parents, it is the final recognition of them as the legal parents of the child that was always intended for them. For the surrogate and her partner, it can feel a little bittersweet – a celebration of the huge achievement they have reached as a team, and an ending of an amazing experience. Regardless of whether there is a hearing, or whether all the parties can attend, it is important to mark the occasion as a team. A special luncheon or dinner to celebrate the final stage of the surrogacy journey and start the next chapter together.

CHAPTER 15

The future

Milestones and rituals

When most people have a child, they celebrate milestones like birthdays and Mother's and Father's Days without having to consult or think about anyone outside their own household or immediate family. The celebrations are for the parents and the child and for the most part, no one else expects to be involved.

In altruistic surrogacy arrangements, the opposite can be true. The baby's birthday is also the anniversary of the surrogate giving birth to the baby and giving the baby to the intended parents. Milestones may mark a variety of different and important occasions for different members of the team on the very same day.

The surrogate may think these occasions are important and special, and not just because they are the celebrations of parenthood and the child. They are important for her too and what she went through being a surrogate.

The surrogate might say that she does not need, or expect,

acknowledgement on these special days. Parents could take her word for it, but they could also acknowledge her anyway. Almost certainly, the surrogate does not want the spotlight on her. She wants the parents to enjoy these events and that is what she has been looking forward to seeing: the family she helped create.

Sometimes these days can be challenging for the parents, perhaps because they bring up the grief of pregnancy losses or infertility. These days can also be challenging for surrogates, and even more so if they feel ignored or forgotten.

So what are the events that might need some celebration or acknowledgment of the surrogate, and how do you do it?

Baby's birthday

Birthdays are a milestone for the birthing mother – it's the anniversary of a life-changing event that she and her family went through. Celebrating the child's birthday is important for intended parents too – it is a celebration of their first year as parents, joyous and challenging as it may have been. My best advice for birthday celebrations is to have one party for the child, and a separate gathering between the parents and the surrogate family to acknowledge the relationship, the journey and the challenges.

Mother's Day

This day is important and can be sensitive for surrogates. She is the birth mother to your child. And while no surrogate is the same, I can tell you that no surrogate has ever been sad to receive a Happy Mother's Day message from her intended parents. Plenty of surrogates have felt forgotten and ignored on Mother's Day. And no doubt, plenty of intended parents have been oblivious to the slight. If you became a mother through surrogacy, your surrogate wants to know that you've thought of her at some point on Mother's Day. If you are a two-dad family that does not celebrate Mother's Day, that is fine. But your surrogate is your child's birth mother, and a simple 'Happy Mother's Day' would help her feel acknowledged and appreciated on this day. It may not seem like much to you, but it is important to her. If you are remembering your mother on Mother's Day, remember your child's birth mother too.

If you are not sure how to acknowledge and show appreciation for your surrogate on these special days, here are a few tips.

Make it a priority. If you know a milestone is coming up, make a plan to include your surrogate or show some appreciation toward her on that day.

It does not need to be elaborate. In fact, surrogates generally do not want elaborate gifts and celebrations.

Keep it simple and heartfelt. The ultimate celebration might be about you and the child, so any acknowledgment or celebration of your surrogate can be as simple as a handwritten card, a bunch of flowers, a photo of the baby or your family. Simple words like 'thank you', 'we love you' and 'we are grateful for what you have done' can be really lovely to receive.

A phone or video call can sometimes be better than a text message. Everyone texts these days. Make her feel special and call her.

If you are having a birthday party, introduce your surrogate to your friends. This is really important. Your friends might not know how to talk to the woman who carried your baby. They have probably never met a surrogate before. Many a surrogate has felt like a circus sideshow at these events. Make sure you use language that you are all comfortable with ('this is our baby's birth mother . . !' or 'this is our surrogate . . !').

Include your surrogate in any speeches or social-media posts. Do not pretend a stork brought you a baby. Acknowledge her existence and show appreciation for what she has done for you. Again, nothing elaborate – simple and heartfelt is all she needs.

You should talk about how to mark these occasions as a team, and do not leave it to the surrogate to raise the issue. She may not have thought about it, but she will feel appreciated if you make the effort to acknowledge her at these important milestones.

Finding happiness beyond surrogacy

Surrogacy can be all-consuming – for the intended parents, and the surrogate family.

But then, surrogacy is not forever. Whether you are a surrogate or the intended parents, there has to be something other than surrogacy, beyond surrogacy, that gives you purpose in your life. And that can be hard, particularly when it has been so intense and consuming. The intended parents have the new purpose of caring for their baby and spending time together as a family. The surrogate, on the other hand, often finds herself at a loose end – no baby to care for, and her good friends are now busy with their baby. So how do we prepare for the time beyond surrogacy? And not just the fourth trimester, which is really about team wellbeing, but beyond that – when we have to try and find ourselves again.

One activity you might want to do is the HAPPY list developed by Clarissa Rayward: www.thehappyfamilylawyer.com. That's health, attitude, passion, purpose and you. In this activity, you list things that you can do to look after your own happiness, beyond surrogacy, and then you can use these lists to develop your own goals to pursue happiness for yourself.

H is for health

We know that physical health is a significant part of overall happiness. What are things that we can do to look after our physical health? It may be as simple as drinking enough water, eating well, getting enough sleep and exercising. Our physical health needs will wax and wane (particularly in relation to pregnancy and post-partum), but if we make it a focus in our lives, good feelings will come from it.

A is for attitude

A positive attitude is crucial to happiness, but it's more than just thinking nice things. We need to look after our emotional wellbeing and that might be through practices such as meditation, mindfulness, and counselling and debriefing. Looking after our emotional health is crucial for surrogacy – for the surrogate, her partner and the intended parents. By looking after ourselves emotionally, we're also looking after each other and the children in our lives, including surro-bub. Never underestimate the stress that surrogacy, infertility, pregnancy, birth and parenting can place us under – and that goes for everyone. It's not just the surrogate who will experience hormonal shifts and emotional challenges in the surrogacy journey, and it is everyone's responsibility to access their own support throughout. Some people find writing in a journal helpful, or yoga practice. For me, running has boosted my physical health and mental wellbeing.

P is for passion

What do you love to do so much that it makes time stand still, that you forget to eat, and nothing else matters? What do you LOVE to do? Are you passionate about animals, gardening, family, the environment? If money was no object, what would you be doing with your time? What are your passions outside of surrogacy? How can you refocus your energy into something else?

P is for purpose

What, besides surrogacy (or the need to use the toilet) gets us out of bed each day? What drives us? What is our WHY? It can be (should be) more than one thing. For many, it might be their children, or family, or helping people. If someone was writing a speech about your life, what would you like them to say about you? 'She worked long hours and never took a day off. . .'? Beyond surrogacy, what is your why? As amazing as surrogacy can be, it's not sustainable to make it our sole purpose. What do we want our lives to be like, beyond surrogacy?

Y is for YOU

This is about finding those things that make you, you. What does your dream life look like? What would you be doing if you were being completely authentic? Who are you, and what do you represent? This should be more than one thing. What are your values, and what can you do to start living by them?

Once you've worked on your HAPPY, the next step is to work on some goals. Goals need to be SMART: specific, measurable, achievable, realistic and timely. Setting and achieving goals is good for emotional wellbeing because we know that we get endorphins when we achieve our goals. Take some time to look at your HAPPY list and set some goals for each aspect.

One year on –
January 2019

Surro-baby, the baby I birthed, turned one in January of 2019. Her dads threw her a party, of course, and like all first birthdays, it was more of an anniversary for the parents than it was a party for the baby. An anniversary of survival, of joy and frustration and tears (hers, theirs and mine!), and love and learning about each other and the journey of parenthood. I'm exhausted just thinking about it and relieved it's not me living it!

So often in the last year I've been asked about my surrogacy journey and specifically about my relationship with the baby and her parents. So much of what we know about surrogacy is what we see in the media, and usually that's based on commercial arrangements overseas. People are curious whether I still see the baby, and whether I have a bond with her and what my relationship is with her parents.

The first days after her birth was a bit of blur of hormones and overwhelming joy and love. The oxytocin was flowing and we (her dads, myself and my partner) were in a of a bubble of love. It was wonderful! It was a bit overwhelming because I felt like there wasn't a guide book for how any of us were supposed to feel or act. I also felt like a bit of a circus act, because we had lots of people sending their well wishes and demanding details of the birth and the surrogacy arrangement, and midwives at the hospital checking in to see whether I was falling apart. We were relieved to leave the hospital and go back to our own comfort zones.

The first weeks were a bit of a mixture of emotions and activity – my partner and I getting on with our home lives, getting the kids ready for kinder and school, him working, and me recovering from birth and expressing milk for the baby. And of course, there were lots of visits with the baby and her dads. I found these weeks a bit strange and, as I like to feel in control, that lack of routine or consistency was a little unsettling. I was rather sad that our surrogacy journey was 'over', and I didn't want it to end because I had had such a great time. I even offered to carry another baby for them immediately. Let's say, the oxytocin ride was amazing, but quite the rollercoaster!

The biggest frustration for me was not being able to drive, and my body not moving the way I wanted it to. I had had a caesarean section, and while I knew intellectually that my body was recovering from major surgery, I was frustrated that I was sore, tired and slow. My youngest child was learning to ride a bike, and I could not move fast enough to keep up. I had to keep reminding myself that I had just had a baby, because part of my brain hadn't caught up to reality. It is one of the amazing things about the body and the mind – of course I knew that I had just had a baby, but it didn't stop me wanting to get back to normal as soon as possible. I had never wanted to care for a newborn again, so why could I not get back to my usual routine?

Over the next few months, there was a gradual weaning process for me and the baby and her dads. In the early weeks we would see each other every day, then every few days, and then once a week, and then once, sometimes twice, a fortnight. They were enjoying their newborn, and I was finding my way as the 'ex' surrogate. What was my role, now that I wasn't pregnant and had no job to do? It was also confusing, and sometimes confronting. Sometimes I resent the impact that surrogacy has had on me and my family, knowing that they got the baby and I got . . . a postpartum body and hair loss. I'm still dealing with the hair loss, which bothers me more than I expected it to.

Even with lots of other things happening in my life, I still had lots of processing and thinking to do about the surrogacy, and the birth, and the baby and her dads. I have access to an amazing surrogacy counsellor, Katrina Hale, who regularly debriefs with me about all this stuff, and I also had lots of support from other surrogates. Having friends who understand the feelings and thoughts is so necessary and appreciated. Traditional surrogacy is all the more complex, and even rarer than gestational surrogacy.

During that time, I was able to put a lot of my creative energy into other things, including creating the *Australian Surrogacy Podcast*, and organising the Surrogacy Sisterhood Day. I also set myself a running goal, to run 10km later that year. Having other things to focus on was really useful.

My relationship with the dads has changed and grown. I

spent a lot of time in the early months second-guessing why they wanted to spend time with me, and sometimes I still do. I worry that they only spend time with me because I gave them a baby, that they feel they have a debt to repay. And they probably do feel indebted to me, but that's not a good foundation for friendship. I remember feeling surprised that they seemed to like spending time with me; perhaps I thought they would stop once the baby was here? Katrina reckons there are two certainties with surrogacy – the surrogate worries that she will be abandoned, and the intended parents worry that she will keep the baby. I admit I was surprised when I fell into the cliché. These days we have a new normal; we spend time together as families and I babysit for her occasionally. I still worry that there is an imbalance of power in our relationship: that they will forever feel they need to express their appreciation and worry that they'll ever offend me. I think most surrogates find the power-imbalance really uncomfortable.

As for my relationship with the baby, it took me a while to realise that it is a journey and not a destination. I remember wanting to know what she would think of me when she is 10, or 15, or 25. Would she know who I am? Would she recognise me? I would see her face and be struck by how familiar she seemed. For some reason, I am surprised by the resemblance she has to me and my kids. Even now, when I see a photo of her in my newsfeed, I draw breath. I know that face! Oh wait, of course I do, it's the baby I birthed. It might be a primal response, which some donors and donor-conceived children also experience when they meet each other. As if we are recognising ourselves in the other person, perhaps. But it took me a while to accept that it is a perpetual journey, that I do not know what my relationship with the baby will look like in the future, and that's OK. I've found comfort in accepting that I have limited control over it, because I do not have all the answers. And at some point she will decide what she needs from me and what our relationship is to be.

These days, I spend time with the baby and her dads regularly. She will know me as Aunty Sarah, and of course she will know her story. But while I recognise her as being from me, and the baby I carried, I do not feel like her parent. I do not feel like I need to take on a parenting role for her. I do not feel bonded to her the way I do to my kids. She looks for her dads when they leave the room – and I find that affirming, because I know her primary attachments are to the people who are her parents, just as we intended. My relationship with her is different; more than an aunt–niece relationship, but not the same as a mother–daughter relationship.

The first birthday and the anniversary of me giving birth feel like two separate events, both worthy of reflection and acknowledgement. 'It's complex' is the best descriptor I can come up with. There is no box that any of this fits in. I felt some peace as we met that milestone – that chapter was closing, while the book was still being written. I have other things to focus on and surrogacy, while sometimes all-consuming, is not a career (unless you are a surrogacy lawyer, of course!).

There have been multiple comments from the dads over the year about how lucky they feel to have her in their lives, and plenty of people reflecting on how lucky she is to have her dads. And I agree on both fronts. But in everything that we went through in the first year, and how much we've shared over the past three years, I must say that I am the luckiest person. I am so privileged to have been a part of this journey and to be a part of her life, and for her dads to have let me be part of theirs.

Surrogacy is incredibly complex, a perpetual journey, and more so than I ever imagined. My life is richer and I am so grateful for it. There is such a special sweetness in participating in creation.

For those intended parents and surrogates and their families, I wish and hope for you to have a positive, amazing surrogacy journey, full of love and laughter and lifelong friendship. Because above all else, your experiences will shape the experience of your future children, and they deserve the very best story.

GLOSSARY

Here are some common terms and abbreviations you will come across in this book and in your surrogacy journey.

IP: intended parent/s

IM: intended mother

IF: intended father

GS: gestational surrogate, a surrogate who carries a baby with an embryo created with an egg from the intended mother or a donor.

TS: traditional surrogate, a surrogate who carries a baby created with her own egg.

Gamete: an egg or sperm.

Parentage order: an order in the State Court that transfers parentage from the birth parents to the intended parents. Parentage Orders are made in Australian surrogacy arrangements.

Parenting order: an order of the Family Court that sets out the arrangements for the care of a child. Some parents may seek a Parenting order after returning to Australia with their child born through international surrogacy.

Surrogacy team: the intended parents and surrogate and her partner that make up the team together.

BEST PRACTICE GUIDELINES FOR
CARE IN SURROGACY

FOR AUSTRALIAN
HEALTHCARE
PROVIDERS

CONTENTS

INTRODUCTION

These guidelines are to assist healthcare practitioners supporting surrogacy pregnancies and births. At all times, the child's best interests are paramount, and the birth mother retains her bodily autonomy. Healthcare providers should acquaint themselves with the legal context of surrogacy arrangements and defer to the parties to assist them to understand the dynamics in each unique relationship.

LANGUAGE

Care providers should discuss the appropriate use of language with the parties to determine the terms they are most comfortable with. The following terms are used in this document:

- *Birth mother*: the pregnant person, also referred to as the surrogate. Some surrogates dislike being referred to as 'birth mother', though the legislation often refers to them in this manner.
- *Birth parents*: the birth mother and their partner.
- *Intended parent/s (IPs)*: the intended parents of the baby, who will take custody of the child from birth. Alternatively, the parties may be referred to as 'intended mother' or 'intended father'. The intended parent/s may be heterosexual or homosexual, coupled or single. The intended parent/s will have qualified for surrogacy prior to conception.
- *Gestational surrogacy (GS)*: This is the most common

type of surrogacy in Australia and involves a surrogate who is not the genetic mother of the child. An egg is provided by the intended mother or a donor, which is fertilised with sperm from an intended father or a donor. The arrangement necessarily involves fertility treatments at an IVF clinic.

- *Traditional surrogacy (TS)*: This is less common in Australia and involves a surrogate who has provided the egg for conception, fertilised with sperm from an intended father or a donor. Whilst traditional surrogacy is legal across Australia (except in the ACT), the parties often conceive without the assistance of an IVF clinic and instead via home insemination.

LEGAL CONTEXT

Altruistic surrogacy is legal in across Australia, except in the Northern Territory where there are currently no surrogacy laws. Surrogacy arrangements have the following elements:

- The arrangement is altruistic; commercial surrogacy is illegal across Australia. Surrogates can be reimbursed for surrogacy-related expenses.
- The parties receive counselling with a qualified surrogacy counsellor prior to entering the arrangement.
- The parties obtain independent legal advice prior to entering the arrangement, and often have a written surrogacy agreement they have signed prior to conception.

- The arrangement is not enforceable.
- The birth mother retains her bodily autonomy throughout pregnancy and birth.
- The birth is registered under the birth parents' names, with the full name chosen by the intended parents. The birth mother's surname can be used on hospital identification documents for the baby. The baby is given the intended parents' chosen surname on the birth registration.
- The birth mother and her partner are the legal parents at the time of the birth. The intended parents will apply for a **parentage order** after the birth, which transfers parentage from the birth parents to the intended parents.

PREGNANCY CARE

The parties should be supported to attend appointments together, with the birth mother's consent. Information should be provided to allow the parties to make decisions together. The birth mother can make the final decision.

The birth mother is entitled to her privacy; medical information about the pregnancy can be shared with the intended parents with the birth mother's consent.

The intended parents should be offered parent-craft and birth classes, and provided with information and supports as appropriate.

BIRTH PLANNING

It is crucial that healthcare providers meet with the birth parents and intended parents to discuss plans for the birth. It is important that the birth mother maintains her bodily autonomy throughout the birth and postpartum.

The birth mother should be supported to have the intended parents present during the birth if that is her preference and circumstances allow. It is important for the birth mother's emotional wellbeing that she can see the intended parents meet the baby, and to remain close by in the first few days. Surrogacy births should also be photographed if practicable and the parties request it.

Arrangements for the birth such as cutting the cord, skin-to-skin, breastfeeding and placenta delivery should be discussed with the parties and information and support provided to allow them to make informed decisions.

FEEDING BABY

The intended parents can provide all care for baby, including feeding, immediately from the moment of birth. This can include:

- The intended parent may induce lactation and feed baby
- The birth mother may breastfeed the baby
- The birth mother may provide expressed colostrum and milk for baby

- The baby may be formula fed
- A combination of the above

The feeding arrangements should be agreed between the parties, and plans will often change throughout the pregnancy and post-birth. The hospital should provide information, support and referrals for all parties to make informed decisions.

POSTNATAL CARE

The birth mother's privacy should be respected, and every effort made to accommodate her in a separate room from the intended parents and baby.

If there are no available rooms for the intended parents to stay, an intended parent should be accommodated to stay in the same room as the birth mother, with the baby.

It is usual for the intended parents to be treated as the parents of the child, subject to any agreement with the birth parents.

The birth mother is not obliged to care for the baby and is unlikely to want to do so. Further, the intended parents should be supported to undertake all care for the baby, including the provision of parent-craft assistance.

The intended parents can care for the baby from the moment of birth. The birth parents may provide consent to any medical treatment of the baby if necessary.

DISCHARGE FROM HOSPITAL & ONGOING CARE

The baby and the birth mother may be discharged together or separately, depending on the circumstances. If there are to be separate discharges, the hospital may seek that the birth parents provide written consent for the intended parents to remain in hospital or leave with the baby.

The intended parents and baby should be provided with home visits as is generally provided to new parents, and referrals for their local child-health nurse. The birth mother should be provided with postnatal checkups and referred to her treating general practitioner as appropriate.

ADDITIONAL RESOURCES

Further information and resources can be found at:
www.sarahjefford.com,
including information about surrogacy pregnancy and birth planning, feeding a surrogacy baby and the importance of surrogacy birth photography. You can contact me on:
sarah@sarahjefford.com.
The Australian Surrogacy Podcast shares stories with surrogates and intended parents and is available at:
www.sarahjefford.com.

ABOUT SARAH

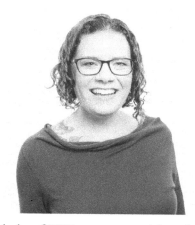

Sarah Jefford is a family and surrogacy lawyer, living in Melbourne with her partner, Troy, and their two sons, Archie and Rafael. Sarah has been a practising lawyer for over 15 years and opened up her own law firm in 2016.

Sarah and Troy conceived their first son, Archie, with the help of IVF treatment. After their second son, Rafael, was born, they considered their family to be complete. Sarah then became an egg donor and donated to several families.

In 2016, Sarah decided to become a surrogate, and she and Troy offered to a same sex male couple in Melbourne. The team underwent counselling and legal advice in accordance with the legal requirements for surrogacy. They were eventually able to conceive a child in a traditional surrogacy arrangement, and Sarah delivered a baby for the two dads in 2018. Sarah, Troy, the parents and all their children are lifelong friends and spend regular time together.

Since opening up her own law firm and becoming an egg donor and a surrogate, Sarah has specialised in surrogacy and donor conception law, or 'family creation' law. She is the only lawyer in Australia to practice exclusively in family creation law, and her clients hail from across Australia.

In 2018, Sarah launched the **Australian Surrogacy Podcast**, sharing stories from surrogates, intended parents and industry professionals, to support others on the surrogacy journey. This podcast celebrated it's 100th episode in 2020.

Sarah speaks regularly on issues of donor conception and altruistic surrogacy. Through her work and advocacy, she promotes best practice altruistic surrogacy arrangements, the best interests of children and the bodily autonomy of women.

Drawing on her experiences as an IVF mum, egg donor, surrogate and lawyer, Sarah wrote *More Than Just a Baby: A Guide to Surrogacy for Intended Parents and Surrogates*.

Sarah says the idea for the book came shortly after she gave birth as a surrogate. 'I felt so many powerful and amazing emotions and wondered whether what I was feeling was normal. I remember thinking 'there really should be a book about this.' So, I wrote that book.'

Sarah is passionate about positive and empowered surrogacy arrangements that focus on the best interests of children, and the longevity of the relationship between the surrogate and the intended parents. 'Surrogacy relationships are the most complex of relationships that we can enter in our lifetime. I want intended parents and surrogates to understand the complexity and gravity of those relationships so they can have a positive, lifelong relationship, well beyond the birth and the legal process.'

Sarah is well respected and recognised for her work in the surrogacy community. In 2019 she was a finalist in the **Thought Leader and Sole Practitioner** categories for the **Women in Law Awards**, and in 2020 she was recognised as a **Finalist Innovator of the Year in the Australian Law Awards**.

Please visit Sarah's website to access additional resources, tips, her Blog and the Australian Surrogacy Podcast:

www.SarahJefford.com

Social Media
Facebook: **facebook.com/sarahjefford**
Instagram: **instagram.com/sarah_surrogacylawyer/**
Linked In: **linkedin.com/in/sarahjefford**
Podcast: **soundcloud.com/australiansurrogacypodcast**

SPEAKING TOPICS

Sarah has spoken on the following topics:

Surrogacy in Australia

Covering topics including:

- The Legal Framework
- Qualifying for surrogacy
- Processes
- Traditional and Gestational Surrogacy
- Surrogacy relationships between birth and intended parents
- Bodily Autonomy, Privacy and Information-Sharing
- The Importance of Surrogacy Birth Photography
- Birth Planning
- Hospital Management of a Surrogacy Birth
- Milk & Feeding a Surrogacy Baby
- The Fourth Trimester
- Best Practice Surrogacy & Ethics
- Parentage Order process and applications
- Ongoing Relationships, Milestones & Celebrations
- How to have a positive surrogacy experience
- How to maintain a positive ongoing relationship

Traditional Surrogacy in Australia

Best Practice Surrogacy in Australia

Donor Conception

Being an egg donor; best practice donor conception; the rights and interests of donor-conceived people

Surrogacy as Motherhood: The Inalienable Right to Choose

Presentation to Melbourne University Law School's Health Law & Ethics Network. Full speech at:
https://sarahjefford.com/surrogacy-as-motherhood/

Altruistic Surrogacy and Ethics

Presentation to the AFCC conference, Sydney 2019
Surrogacy, donor conception and ethics – balancing the best interests of the child, the autonomy of the surrogate and the interests of the intended parents

Surrogacy in Australia: Considerations for Healthcare Providers

Presentation to the Australian College of Midwives, March 2020

ACKNOWLEDGEMENTS

The years since travelling through the world of infertility and IVF, motherhood, egg donation and surrogacy have taught me that we are nothing without our village. *More Than Just a Baby* is further proof that it not only does it take a village to raise a child, but sometimes it takes a village to write a book.

First and foremost, I must thank my partner Troy, who has been my quiet and consistent supporter and champion. And our children Archie and Raf, who provide me with endless creative inspiration, thank you for keeping me in the moment.

Of course, thanks must go to my intended parents Mike and Nate, who allowed me the privilege of becoming part of their family and who light me up every day. This book would not have been written, of course, were it not for the birth of their daughter Darcey, and I am grateful for the chance to bring her into the world and watch her grow.

I would be nothing without the unending support of the Surrogacy Sisterhood, who truly understand what it is to carry a baby for someone else and that validate our shared experiences.

Thanks must also go to the Australian surrogacy community, intended parents and surrogates who have generously shared their journeys with me.

A very special thank you to Katrina Hale, psychologist, who's wealth of knowledge and expertise contributed not only to my own personal growth, but to my understanding of the surrogacy experience. Katrina also kindly read and reviewed the book and I'm grateful for her contribution.

Sarah Nowoweiski has been my infertility, pregnancy, egg donation and surrogacy counsellor over the years, and I now have the privilege of calling her a friend. A big thank you, for now also being a book reviewer and supporter.

Heartfelt thanks to my first readers and reviewers, Phillipa Ross, Heidi Jensen, Amanda Meehan, Anna McKie, Jarrad and Michael Duggan-Tierney and Ben Sayer. I am so grateful for the enthusiasm, curiosity and support from so many people, and the book is all the better for the contributions of other people who share my passion.

CPSIA information can be obtained
at www.ICGtesting.com
Printed in the USA
BVHW031700290922
648311BV00011B/413